Introduction to Epidemiology

Understanding Public Health Series

Series editors: Nicki Thorogood and Rosalind Plowman, London School of Hygiene & Tropical Medicine

Throughout the world, recognition of the importance of public health to sustainable, safe, and healthy societies is growing. The achievements of public health in nineteenth-century Europe were for much of the twentieth century overshadowed by advances in personal care, in particular in-hospital care. Now, with the dawning of a new century, there is increasing understanding of the inevitable limits of individual health care and of the need to complement such services with effective public health strategies. Major improvements in people's health will come from controlling communicable diseases, eradicating environmental hazards, improving people's diets, and enhancing the availability and quality of effective health care. To achieve this, every country needs a cadre of knowledgeable public health practitioners with social, political, and organizational skills to lead and bring about changes at international, national, and local levels.

This is one of a series of books that provides a foundation for those wishing to join in and contribute to the twenty-first-century regeneration of public health, helping to put the concerns and perspectives of public health at the heart of policy-making and service provision. While each book stands alone, together they provide a comprehensive account of the three main aims of public health: protecting the public from environmental hazards, improving the health of the public, and ensuring high-quality health services are available to all. Some of the books focus on methods, others on key topics. They have been written by staff at the London School of Hygiene & Tropical Medicine with considerable experience of teaching public health to students from low-, middle-, and high-income countries. Much of the material has been developed and tested with postgraduate students both in face-to-face teaching and through distance learning.

The books are designed for self-directed learning. Each chapter has explicit learning objectives, key terms are highlighted, and the text contains many activities to enable the reader to test their own understanding of the ideas and material covered. Written in a clear and accessible style, the series will be essential reading for students taking postgraduate courses in public health and will also be of interest to public health practitioners and policy-makers.

Titles in the series

Analytical models for decision making: Colin Sanderson and Reinhold Gruen
Conflict and health: Natasha Howard, Egbert Sondorp, and Annemarie Ter Veen (eds.)
Controlling communicable disease: Norman Noah
Economic analysis for management and policy: Stephen Jan, Lilani Kumaranayake, Jenny Roberts, Kara Hanson, and Kate Archibald
Economic evaluation: Julia Fox-Rushby and John Cairns (eds.)
Environmental epidemiology: Paul Wilkinson (ed.)
Environmental health policy: Megan Landon and Tony Fletcher
Environment, health and sustainable development, Second Edition: Emma Hutchinson and Sari Kovats
Financial management in health services: Reinhold Gruen and Anne Howarth
Health care evaluation, Second Edition: Carmen Tsang and David Cromwell
Health promotion theory, Second Edition: Liza Cragg, Maggie Davies, and Wendy MacDowall (eds.)
Health promotion practice, Second Edition: Will Nutland and Liza Cragg (eds.)
Introduction to health economics, Second Edition: Lorna Guinness and Virginia Wiseman (eds.)
Issues in public health, Second Edition: Fiona Sim and Martin McKee (eds.)
Making health policy, Second Edition: Kent Buse, Nicholas Mays, and Gill Walt
Managing health services: Nick Goodwin, Reinhold Gruen, and Valerie Iles
Medical anthropology: Robert Pool and Wenzel Geissler
Principles of social research, Second Edition: Mary Alison Durand and Tracey Chantler (eds.)
Public health in history: Virginia Berridge, Martin Gorsky, and Alex Mold
Sexual health: A public health perspective: Kay Wellings, Kirstin Mitchell, and Martine Collumbien (eds.)
Understanding health services, Second Edition: Ipek Gürol-Urgancı, Fiona Campbell, and Nick Black

Forthcoming titles

Applied communicable disease control: Liza Cragg, Will Nutland, and R. Gregory Thomas-Reilly

Introduction to Epidemiology

Third edition

Ilona Carneiro

 Open University Press

Open University Press
McGraw-Hill Education
8th Floor, 338 Euston Road
London
England
NW1 3BH

email: enquiries@openup.co.uk
world wide web: www.openup.co.uk

and Two Penn Plaza, New York, NY 10121-2289, USA

First Published 2005
Second Edition Published 2011
First Published in this third edition 2017
First published 2017

A catalogue record of this book is available from the British Library

ISBN-13: 978-0-335-24317-4
ISBN-10: 0-33-524317-7
eISBN: 978-0-335-24318-1

Library of Congress Cataloging-in-Publication Data
CIP data applied for

Typeset by Transforma Pvt. Ltd., Chennai, India

Printed and bound in Great Britain by Bell & Bain Ltd, Glasgow

Fictitious names of companies, products, people, characters and/or data that may be used herein (in case studies or in examples) are not intended to represent any real individual, company, product or event.

MIX
Paper from responsible sources
FSC® C007785

For Enrique, Ariana, and Alesia Marin

Contents

List of figures and tables

Figures

Tables

Preface

This book represents a thorough revision of the second edition. Chapter 1 now includes a section on the historical development of epidemiology as a discipline, and Chapter 5 includes material on correlation coefficients. The structure of the book has been modified to include a new chapter on descriptive epidemiology (Chapter 6), combining some of the previous text on standardization and routine data with a new section on outbreak investigation. The previous chapters on analytical studies (ecological, cross-sectional, cohort, and case-control) have now been combined into one (Chapter 7). A new final chapter has been added to include more general exercises and an activity on the 2016 Zika outbreak to integrate some of the different concepts learned.

The examples and activities have been revised and updated to maintain a wide range of current global health issues. The number of activities has been increased to help readers test their understanding of the material as they progress through the book. Several diagrams have been designed and more figures have been added to help visualization of difficult concepts. All tables and figures in this book were designed and prepared by Ilona Carneiro, unless stated otherwise.

Acknowledgements

The author wishes to thank all colleagues who developed the original lectures and teaching materials at the London School of Hygiene & Tropical Medicine, especially Lucianne Bailey, Katerina Vardulaki, Julia Langham, and Daniel Chandramohan who wrote the first edition; those who taught the LSHTM Zika online course; Mark Taylor and Sue Cliffe (module organizers) for reviewing draft chapters; Ros Plowman and Nicki Thorogood (series editors) and Natasha Howard (second edition co-author), who fully reviewed this third edition.

I am grateful to the students of the Public Health distance learning Basic Epidemiology module for challenging me to improve the material over the years, and to all the students who piloted the activities in this edition, especially Patricia Lledó Weber, Sepideh Bagheri Nejad, and Stamatina Kambanarou, who gave very useful feedback on the draft manuscript.

Overview of the book

Introduction

This book is intended for self-directed learning. It provides a summary of the main concepts and methods of epidemiology as a foundation for further study. It will also introduce more advanced epidemiological and statistical concepts to broaden understanding. After completing the book, you should be able to apply basic epidemiological methods and critically interpret the epidemiological findings of others.

Why study epidemiology?

Epidemiology is integral to public health. Whether your interest is in clinical or public health medicine, the study of epidemiology is key to improving health. Neither clinical nor public health practice can be based on experience alone. They must be informed by scientific evidence. Understanding the appropriateness of different research methods is essential to critical appraisal of the evidence presented in scientific literature. The ability to distinguish between strong and poor evidence is fundamental to promoting evidence-informed health care. This ability is important for all those who work in health-related areas, including health economists, health policy analysts, and health services managers. Epidemiology is central to clinical research, disease prevention, health promotion, health protection, and health services research.

Epidemiology offers rigorous methods to study the distribution, causation, and prevention of poor health in populations. It enables a better understanding of health and the factors that influence it at the individual and population level. Epidemiological methods are also used to investigate the usefulness of preventive and therapeutic interventions, and the coverage of healthcare services. The purpose of epidemiology is to use these methods and the resulting data to improve health and survival.

Structure of the book

This book is structured around the basic concepts, practices, and applications of epidemiology and uses the conceptual framework of the basic epidemiology module taught face-to-face at the London School of Hygiene & Tropical Medicine. It is based on material presented in lectures and seminars, which has been adapted for independent learning.

Chapters 1–4 discuss the principles of epidemiology and introduce strategies for measuring the frequency of health outcomes, associations, and impact of exposures, and evaluating whether an association is causal. Chapters 5–8 focus on practical aspects of epidemiological research, including issues of study design and data collection, and the strengths and weaknesses of each of the principal epidemiological study designs. Chapters 9 and 10 consider the application of epidemiology for prevention strategies and for surveillance, monitoring, and evaluation. Finally, Chapter 11 aims to integrate the scientific knowledge learned and apply it to contemporary health issues.

Each chapter includes:

- an overview;
- a list of learning objectives;
- a range of activities;
- a concluding summary; and
- feedback on the activities.

Words presented in **bold** are described in the Glossary. You may find the index at the end of the book useful for finding specific items of information that you are unsure of or wish to review.

Guidance notes for activities

We recommend that you attempt the activities as they appear in the text, and refer to the preceding explanatory text if you find a question unclear or difficult. You should complete the whole of each activity before reading the relevant feedback at the end of each chapter, as this will help you to assess your understanding of the material presented. Written answers are not always exhaustive, but provide an indication of an acceptable response. You will sometimes provide a different written response to that given in the feedback – this does not necessarily mean that you have misunderstood the material, as some responses are subjective and may depend on your perspective or previous experience. Additional information, which is given for your understanding but not expected as part of your answer, is shown in square brackets [...].

As is usual in epidemiology, many activities will include a numerical calculation and require interpretation of results. The required mathematical skills are basic, but may require the use of a calculator. Proportions (e.g. 0.20) can be presented as percentages by multiplying by 100 (i.e. $0.20 \times 100 = 20\%$). Decimals should generally be rounded to two decimal places (e.g. 0.148 reported as 0.15), while statistical probability values are usually rounded to three decimal places (e.g. $P = 0.0025$ reported as $P = 0.003$). It is important not to round numbers until the very end of a mathematical operation, to avoid the accumulation of error due to rounding and to maintain precision.

SECTION 1

Principles of epidemiology

Understanding epidemiology 1

Overview

Epidemiology is fundamental to public health. It employs rigorous quantitative methods to study the health of *populations* rather than individuals. Epidemiological methods are used to identify the causes of poor health, measure the strength of associations between causes and outcomes, evaluate interventions to improve health, and monitor changes in population health over time. The study of epidemiology provides an essential part of the evidence base for appropriate public health policy, planning, and practice. This chapter introduces you to the purpose and key approaches of epidemiological research and practice.

Learning objectives

When you have completed this chapter, you should be able to:

- identify the main uses of epidemiology
- describe the role of epidemiology in society
- recognize the complex factors involved in the study of causality
- list the basic study designs used in epidemiology

What is epidemiology?

Epidemiology is *the study* of the distribution and determinants of health states or events in specified populations, and *the application* of this study to control health problems (adapted from Porta and International Epidemiological Association, 2008).

Epidemiology is a form of 'detective work', summarized by answering the 'Five Ws':

1. *What* is the **outcome** of interest? Health states or events usually refer to infection, illness, disability or death but may equally refer to a positive outcome such as survival.
2. *Who* is at risk? Some individuals or populations are more likely to develop the outcome, and the characteristics that determine this are known as

risk factors (e.g. poverty) or protective factors (e.g. vaccination), depending on whether they result in a negative or positive health outcome.

3. *Where* is it seen? Outcomes may vary by country or region because of environmental conditions (e.g. pollution) or population differences (e.g. genetics or diet; see *Who?* above).

4. *When* does it happen? Some health events may be seasonal (e.g. pollen allergies) or may vary over years (e.g. measles), increasing or decreasing in relation to a risk factor.

5. *Why* does it happen? In addition to describing the distribution of health outcomes by time, place, and personal or population characteristics, epidemiologists also investigate potential reasons for an association between a risk factor and an outcome, and try to understand the underlying cause of the outcome.

Epidemiological research also involves the testing of preventive interventions (e.g. vaccines, improved hygiene) and therapeutic interventions (e.g. medicines, surgery) to improve health and survival. An intervention may be evaluated either under ideal (research-controlled) conditions to assess its **efficacy** or during routine delivery to assess its **effectiveness**.

After collecting all the epidemiological evidence, we can use it to improve health. The identification of risk factors and protective interventions, and quantification of their effects, is key to informing action. Knowledge of the distribution and time-trends of outcomes, risk factors, and intervention coverage may be used for advocacy, for health promotion, and to inform public health policy and practice.

A brief history of epidemiology

To understand the role of epidemiology in society today, we will review its development as a scientific discipline, highlighting some of the key figures who have advanced our knowledge and practice.

Important early figures in epidemiology

Hippocrates (460–375 BC), a Greek physician, wrote in the fifth century BC: 'Whoever wishes to investigate medicine properly, should proceed thus: in the first place to consider the seasons, and what effects each of them produces . . . We must also consider the qualities of the waters . . . and the mode in which the inhabitants live, and what are their pursuits, whether they are fond of drinking & eating to excess, and given to indolence, or are fond of exercise & labour' (Hippocrates, 2015). His advice to observe the climate, environment, and population behaviours still forms the basis of most epidemiological investigation into the causes of outcomes.

John Graunt (1620–1674) was an English salesman who, more than 2000 years later, developed a more systematic approach. Repeated **outbreaks** of the plague in Europe between the fourteenth and seventeenth centuries led to the development of weekly registers of deaths in London, to monitor the impact of the plague. Graunt used these *Bills of Mortality* to analyse patterns of births and deaths in 1662, establishing him as one of the first demographers (Rothman, 1996). He was the first to report that more boys than girls are born, presenting one of the first **life-tables**. Graunt used these routinely collected data to describe new diseases and report on the frequencies of various causes of death, summarizing the numbers by season, year, and geographic area.

Bernardino Ramazzini (1633–1714) was an Italian physician who, between 1700 and 1713, published his observations on the diseases of workers, and is considered the 'father of occupational medicine'. His systematic study and insights into the effects of occupational exposure to chemical or physical agents, as well as repetitive movements and posture, are still relevant today (Ramazzini, 2001). He also proposed that breast cancer (known in those days as 'nun's disease') might be related to the nuns' celibate lifestyle – more than 250 years before the association between breast cancer and reproductive history was shown.

James Lind (1716–1794) was a Scottish military surgeon who noticed high mortality from scurvy (now known to be caused by vitamin C deficiency) among sailors. In 1747, he compared different treatments for sailors suffering from scurvy and observed that eating oranges and lemons produced the best outcome. He reported this first ever controlled **clinical trial** (Bhatt, 2010), and advanced the practice of preventive medicine.

Pierre-Charles-Alexandre Louis (1787–1872) was a French physician who made detailed clinical observations and conducted autopsies of patients in Paris. He applied a standardized method of data collection and analysis at a group level, which developed into today's clinical epidemiology (Morabia, 1996).

✎ Activity 1.1

Until the nineteenth century, bloodletting (the release of blood by cutting a vein or applying leeches) was an accepted treatment for inflammatory diseases and was widespread in England and France. Louis decided to determine whether it worked by reviewing his clinical records of 77 patients with pneumonia. Table 1.1 shows the results of his study, comparing the numbers of days of illness among those who survived and the numbers that died, by day of first bleeding in relation to the start of symptoms.

Describe what Louis' results show and briefly interpret his findings.

Table 1.1 Duration of illness and number of deaths by day of first bleeding

Day of first bleeding	Number of subjects	Average duration of illness (days)	Number that died
1–4	41	17.8	18
5–9	36	20.8	9

Source: Adapted from Morabia (1996).

William Farr (1807–1883), an English physician influenced by Louis, was put in charge of the first national system for the registration of births and deaths, developed to record property transfer in England and Wales in 1836 (Lilienfeld, 2007). Farr then used these data to develop a system of disease classification and compile annual reports on causes of death and mortality by occupation, laying the groundwork for medical statistics.

John Snow (1813–1858), an English physician, is considered one of the fathers of modern epidemiology because of his work on the devastating cholera outbreaks in London between 1848 and 1855. He undertook detailed investigations, generated a new hypothesis, analysed the data he collected, and instigated a public health intervention (Snow, 1936). Prior to development of the 'germ theory of disease', which identified that some diseases are caused by microorganisms, the common belief was that cholera and bubonic plague were the result of a miasma (an unhealthy or poisonous air). Snow's case studies of cholera led him to discount the miasma theory and identify appropriate preventive measures such as personal hygiene and provision of clean water, decades before the *Vibrio cholera* bacterium in water was identified as the causative agent in 1883.

Snow realized that some of the water-pump wells were contaminated with sewage. He used the national registration system to collect details of all cholera deaths in an outbreak in Soho in 1854. He plotted the geographical locations of all cases and went door-to-door to collect information on daily habits. From these he identified a specific public water pump as being the most likely source of the outbreak. He convinced the local authorities to remove the pump-handle, which is now considered a symbol of public health intervention (Figure 1.1).

After the outbreak subsided, the authorities replaced the pump-handle as the idea of faecal-oral disease transmission was considered too disgusting. William Farr's studies had suggested that cholera was associated with altitude, as there were more cases at lower elevations, which supported his belief in the miasma theory. The association with elevation was in fact due to those living downstream consuming water that had been contaminated upstream. This shows the complexity of identifying causation, and the difficulty of influencing public health practice. It wasn't until cholera returned

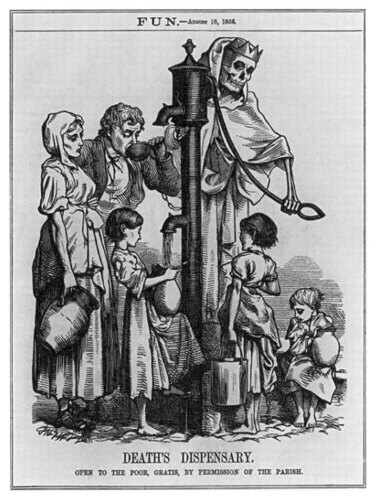

FUN.—August 18, 1866.

DEATH'S DISPENSARY.
OPEN TO THE POOR, GRATIS, BY PERMISSION OF THE PARISH.

Figure 1.1 Caricature by George Pinwell after Snow's theory of contaminated water as the source of cholera came to be accepted

Source: Fun magazine (1866).

to London in 1866, after Snow had died, that Farr realized Snow had been correct and campaigned for sewerage and safe water (Richards, 1983).

Joseph Goldberger (1874–1929), an American physician and epidemiologist, is known for his work on pellagra, a skin disease. In the early 1900s, it was thought that an infectious agent was the cause of pellagra. However, during an **epidemic** in the American South, Goldberger observed that staff from mental hospitals and orphanages did not contract the disease. This led him to suspect a nutritional deficiency as the cause, and he experimented with an enriched feeding programme in selected wards of a mental asylum, with other wards acting as an unplanned control group, and showed a rapid decline in the recurrence of pellagra in the treated group. To prove his case, he then boldly experimented on 11 consenting prison inmates, to show that an imposed poor diet could cause pellagra! He also undertook a community-based study comparing the diets in poor households with and without pellagra, once more showing a clear association between diet and disease. Goldberger's methodical approach to investigating the cause, from basic observations to laboratory experiments, intervention trials, and community studies, highlighted the link with poverty and malnutrition, but he died before the precise cause of pellagra was identified to be a deficiency in niacin, or vitamin B3, in 1937 (Elmore and Feinstein, 1994).

Twentieth-century developments in epidemiology

Once Louis Pasteur and Robert Koch had formally identified microbial agents in the late nineteenth century, it made it easier to identify the causes of many diseases. Patrick Manson discovered that many tropical infectious diseases required a vector (an intermediate organism) for person-to-person transmission, and this work became the basis of vector control interventions in tropical medicine. The study of epidemiology focused on specific infectious causes, and public health intervention shifted from improving sanitation and general living conditions towards preventing individuals from getting infected or preventing the infected from getting sick or dying. The emphasis was on 'infectious disease epidemiology', and clinical trials of vaccines and drug treatments in a patient-centred approach.

With the development of vaccines in the late nineteenth century and antibiotics in the early twentieth century, infectious diseases began to decline in more economically developed countries. Attention shifted to 'chronic disease epidemiology' as mortality from lung cancer and heart disease began to increase, and cancer registries were set up in the USA and Denmark. The discipline of epidemiology was included in clinical training and developed as a postgraduate specialization. Epidemiological methods were developed and applied with increasing success.

Janet Lane-Claypon (1877–1967) was an English physician and a pioneer of many of the epidemiological methods we still use today. In 1912, she reported the first retrospective **cohort study** when she compared a large number of babies who had been fed boiled cows' milk with a similar number of babies fed human breast milk, and showed that the latter group gained more weight. She described the concept of **confounding** and tried to adjust for socio-economic differences. In 1926, she reported a **case-control study** where she compared 500 hospitalized women with breast cancer with the same number of controls, and identified several important risk factors (Winkelstein, 2006). These rigorous methodological developments paved the way for many more epidemiological advances.

In 1950, Richard Doll and Austin Bradford Hill published a large and rigorous case-control study (Doll and Hill, 1950), which together with three other case-control studies highlighted the link between smoking and lung cancer. Subsequent long-term cohort studies confirmed this association. The Framingham Heart Study started in Massachusetts in 1948 as a long-term cardiovascular cohort study to follow 6000 individuals over 30 years. Over the following decades, it showed the effects of high blood pressure, high cholesterol, smoking, obesity, and physical inactivity on heart disease (Boston University, 2016). These and subsequent studies changed the focus of epidemiology to the study of multiple risk factors for chronic diseases. Many health issues gained media attention, and the public became familiar with the concept of 'risk factors' and with taking responsibility for their own health. However, the focus of epidemiological investigations continued to be the risk to the individual, rather than the population.

Late twentieth-century developments

Towards the end of the twentieth century, infectious disease epidemiology interests shifted to the public health arena, with a focus on vaccine-preventable diseases. The Expanded Program on Immunization (EPI) was established in 1974, with the aim of protecting infants throughout the world with life-saving vaccines. One of the greatest achievements of public health was the eradication of smallpox in 1980. Smallpox had mostly disappeared from industrialized countries by the 1940s due to vaccination programmes, but with the development of a heat-stable vaccine in the 1950s, the World Health Organization (WHO) could attempt global elimination. The programme relied on understanding the epidemiology of small-pox, as well as on trained field epidemiologists to undertake surveillance programmes. Following this success, disease prevention and health promotion were given greater emphasis throughout the world (Henderson, 1987).

However, the confidence that infectious diseases had been conquered was soon undermined as new infections emerged. The human immuno-deficiency virus (HIV) associated with acquired immunodeficiency syndrome (AIDS) was identified in the United States in the 1980s, while a variant form of Creutzfeldt-Jakob Disease (vCJD) associated with the bovine spongiform encephalitis (BSE) outbreak in cattle in Britain appeared in the 1990s. The heavy reliance of twentieth-century medicine on the 'magic bullets' of anti-infective drugs and insecticides, and their consequent overuse, led to the evolution of resistance. This in turn led to a re-emergence of previously controlled diseases such as tuberculosis, malaria, and dengue.

In the mid- to late twentieth century, epidemiological methods were applied to the study of a wider range of outcomes, including injury, psychiatric and neurological disorders. Rather than expressing causality in purely biological terms, epidemiologists began to describe a causal web of biological, social, and environmental factors that interact. Advances in statistical techniques further enabled multi-level modelling to take account of these complex interactions, and to detect smaller individual effects of risk factors.

The field of 'genetic epidemiology' developed and evolved rapidly. Early studies compared the risk of disease in groups of relatives to the risk in the **general population**, to identify what **proportion** could be attributed to genetics. This 'familial aggregation' is complicated by similarities in the social factors discussed above, and one way of refining this was to compare the risk of disease by degree of relatedness. Several studies compared the risks in siblings and in identical and non-identical twins. Once a genetic component had been established, studies looked to identify the mechanisms by which these risks were inherited. For example, the haemoglobin disorders of thalassaemia and sickle cell anaemia were described and family studies led to an interest in molecular pathology. Subsequent innovations in molecular biology led to an understanding of molecular-level risk factors for disease, while sequencing of the human genome between 1990 and 2000 enabled the identification of genetic determinants of disease. This indicated that for many diseases there is likely to be a complex interaction of multiple genes of small effect, gene–gene interactions, and gene–environment interactions, such as social factors that also tend to be shared within a family (Kaprio, 2000).

A new discipline of 'social epidemiology' emerged, re-focusing epidemiological investigation on the population context and on social conditions (as Snow and Goldberger had done). Epidemiologists worked with social scientists and health economists to study the effects of the social determinants of health, such as social class, income distribution, ethnicity, gender, and discrimination (Honjo, 2004).

The field of 'health economics' developed from the study of financing and delivery of health services, and of how access to these services and other economic factors affected individual and population health. This field continues to grow and to inform decision-makers as they consider how best to use limited resources to improve public health. Health economists also analyse the decision-making processes of individuals and policy-makers that may affect health outcomes.

Many improvements in population health can be achieved by changes in individual risk behaviours or in the availability of treatments and interventions. However, in some cases epidemiological evidence needs to be translated into 'health policy', or 'decisions, plans and actions undertaken to achieve specific healthcare goals within a society' (World Health Organization, 2016d). This helps to outline priorities, build consensus, and inform people, as demonstrated by national vaccination policies. Sometimes these policies are enforced by legislation, to enact change at a population level. Such laws started in the nineteenth century with the Public Health Acts to improve sanitation and living conditions in the UK, and with universal vaccination against smallpox in England. Key examples of public health legislation in the twentieth century include the requirement for childhood vaccinations before attending school in many countries, and more recently banning smoking in workplaces and public places in several countries.

Another field which has received increasing attention is the role of 'ethics' (the moral code that guides behaviour) in epidemiology and public health

(Coughlin, 2006). As in clinical medicine, ethical guidelines have been developed for the conduct and reporting of epidemiological research studies. These have dealt with minimizing risk and providing benefits to study participants, obtaining informed consent, maintaining confidentiality, and avoiding or disclosing conflicts of interest. The implementation of public health policy and legislation raises many concerns about balancing individual freedoms with protecting public welfare, especially in relation to quarantine and surveillance for infectious diseases. There are also concerns about fair distribution of, and equitable access to, public health resources.

What are the challenges we face today?

There are health disparities between countries and within societies. In areas of poverty, many preventable diseases still occur due to poor hygiene and lack of access to vaccines or medicines. As standards of living improve, attention focuses more on the role of environmental pollution and lifestyle factors (e.g. diet, exercise) on the growing burden of chronic diseases such as cancer, heart disease, obesity, and diabetes. Population ageing across the world is resulting in a new profile of health concerns, such as increasing dementia and disability.

With increasing migration and widespread international travel, there is a greater opportunity for the global spread of emerging infections, such as SARS, bird flu, swine flu, and Ebola. Climate and habitat change are also affecting the geographical distribution of vector-borne diseases, such as dengue, Chikungunya, and Zika. Armed conflicts and natural disasters result in displaced populations and the breakdown of health services, with consequent negative health effects.

The new millennium has also been marked by rapid progress in science and technology. Advances in information technology have resulted in large and complex sets of data ('big data') from medical records, genomics, etc., and increases in computing power enable increasingly sophisticated statistical analyses of these. The use of mobile technologies for geographical mapping, data entry, processing, and even diagnostics, is changing the way that epidemiologists collate and share data. As we saw from the historical examples, producing the evidence is not enough to generate change. There is need for effective communication of findings to decision-makers and to the public; the mass media and social media are playing an increasingly important role in this.

With the challenges of the twenty-first century, there is a continuing and important role for epidemiological research to identify health threats and determine how we can improve health more equitably. Technological advances will bring many advantages, and epidemiology will evolve to make the most of this changing landscape. Epidemiology is now a multidisciplinary field, involving cooperation with molecular biologists, clinicians, statisticians, social scientists, health economists, health policy experts, and many more. We have many more tools and skills at our disposal, and we can use these to provide the evidence base for effective public health solutions.

The study of epidemiology

As we have seen from the historical examples, there are different approaches to the study of epidemiology. These can be categorized as **observational studies**, where the exposure has already been assigned by nature, circumstances or behaviour, or as **intervention studies**, where the investigator assigns the exposure. Observational studies can further be divided into descriptive or analytical studies, with the latter always having a comparison group.

Descriptive epidemiology

Descriptive epidemiology provides information on the distribution of health outcomes by age, population type, geography, and/or over time. This may be done through a **survey** or by following a population over time (Figure 1.2). Sources of descriptive data include routine monitoring such as registers of births and deaths (as used by Graunt and by Farr), notification systems of specific diseases or adverse treatment reactions, and hospital or clinic records. Population censuses also provide data on births, deaths, and a variety of risk factors such as age and gender. There is an overlap with demography, which involves research on changes in the size, structure, and distribution of human populations. Population health surveys have evolved to provide information on the use of health services, coverage of interventions, and frequency of specific outcomes.

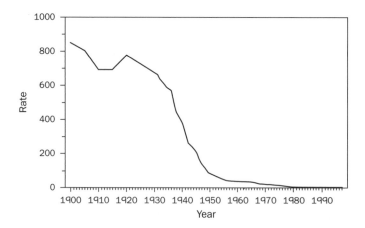

Figure 1.2 Maternal mortality rate per 100,000 live births, by year in the USA, 1900–1997
Source: Centers for Disease Control and Prevention (1999).

Cause and effect

Analytical epidemiology aims to investigate which risk factor – from here on termed '**exposure**' – may be responsible for causing an effect on health – termed 'outcome'. By identifying the exposure and determining why it leads to the outcome, we may be able to intervene and improve health. However, identifying the cause of an outcome is not simple, as it requires us to know what would have happened if there had been no exposure. This is called the **counterfactual** and cannot be observed, as the outcome has already occurred. In epidemiology, we therefore identify a comparison group to represent this 'counterfactual' alternative reality, and call this the **unexposed** group. This comparison between the two groups (exposed and unexposed) to quantify any difference in outcome is the basis of analytical epidemiology.

Relating a causative agent or risk factor to an outcome of interest is not always simple. It is known as inferring **causality** (see Chapter 4). For an association to be causal, the exposure must occur before the outcome. Inferring causality is a complex process because there may be several risk factors that contribute in different ways to the outcome. These can be described in terms of sufficient and component causes (Rothman and Greenland, 2005).

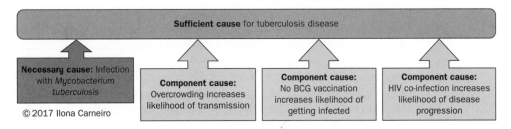

Figure 1.3 Example of sufficient cause for tuberculosis disease

Sufficient cause refers to the set of factors or conditions that can produce an outcome. The factors that comprise the sufficient cause are called **component causes**, and contribute to the outcome occurring. A component cause that is essential for the outcome to occur is known as a **necessary cause**, for example tuberculosis cannot occur without *Mycobacterium tuberculosis*. Figure 1.3 shows that while tuberculosis will not develop in the absence of *M. tuberculosis*, exposure and even infection is insufficient to cause disease on its own. Other component causes can facilitate this process, but are not necessary to cause disease.

Necessary causes include:

- infectious agents such as viruses, bacteria or parasites;
- environmental agents such as the rays of the Sun or allergens (e.g. pollen, dust-mites);
- industrial agents such as chemicals (e.g. nicotine) or sources of radiation (e.g. mobile phones);
- genetic factors such as chromosomal abnormalities;
- physical factors such as violence or car accidents; and
- psychological factors such as stress or abuse.

A single necessary cause is rarely sufficient to produce the outcome. For example, some people may be infected with *M. tuberculosis* without developing tuberculosis, because other component causes such as immune status or concurrent infections (e.g. HIV) will determine their susceptibility to the disease. While this may make epidemiological investigation of causality more difficult to untangle, it works to our advantage in public health, as it means that there are often several points at which we can intervene to reduce the likelihood of an outcome.

Component causes may influence an individual's contact with (exposure to), or their response to, a necessary cause. Environmental factors tend to affect exposure and may be physical (e.g. climate, altitude), biological (e.g. vectors that transmit an agent) or structural (e.g. crowding, sanitation). Human factors affect both exposure and response and include age, sex, ethnicity, behaviour, genetics, and nutritional and immunological status. These environmental and human factors also interact, making the whole process even more complex. For example, people living in conditions of poor sanitation will have greater exposure to the poliovirus because transmission is mainly via faecal contamination. Children will be at greater risk of infection than adults because of potentially poorer sanitary practices and because of their lack of natural immunity or incomplete immunization.

As causation is often the result of the interaction of multiple factors, a cause does not need to be either necessary or sufficient for its removal to result in disease prevention (Rothman and Greenland, 2005). For example, phenylketonuria (PKU) is a rare genetic condition that is present from birth. The body is unable to break down a substance called phenylalanine, which builds up in the blood and brain, and can cause intellectual and developmental disabilities. Dietary restrictions can keep phenylalanine concentrations low and prevent disability, even though the necessary cause (the genetic mutation) has not been removed. An understanding of the component causes is therefore a sound basis for public health intervention. While there may be a complex of causes at the individual level, it may be easier to identify the most important necessary cause by looking at the population level.

As you may have realized, depending on the perspective taken, a cause could also be considered an outcome for the purpose of epidemiological

investigation. For example, human immunodeficiency virus (HIV) is a necessary cause of acquired immunodeficiency syndrome (AIDS). However, we
might want to consider HIV infection as an outcome, and identify the
necessary cause as either unprotected sex with an infected individual or
contact with contaminated needles. This leads us to consider other risk
factors that might increase the likelihood of HIV infection, such as multiple
sexual partners, the sharing of intravenous needles or poor safety practices in health facilities. While these other risk factors may be component
causes, they are not necessary causes. A person may become infected
through only one unprotected sexual contact, while another person with
multiple sexual partners may not become infected.

Analytical epidemiology

The main approach to investigating causal relationships is by comparing
outcomes in different exposure groups, through analytical and intervention
studies. An epidemiological investigation starts with the development of a
hypothesis, which takes the form of a proposed association that can be
tested. For example, 'smokers are at a higher risk of lung cancer than
non-smokers'. A study will then aim to find out whether there is sufficient or
insufficient evidence to support this hypothesis, and to quantify the strength
of any association between the exposure and outcome. The study designs
that form the core of modern epidemiological research are introduced briefly
below, and will be considered in more detail in Chapters 5–10.

Activity 1.3

John Snow believed that contaminated water was the source of the
1848 cholera outbreaks in London, so he analysed the number of
cholera deaths according to their water supply (Snow, 1936). Private
companies responsible for London's water supply obtained their water
directly from the River Thames and supplied drinking water through their
own networks of pipes. Sewage was also emptied directly into the River
Thames, and companies' filtration processes were unlikely to have been
adequate.

The two major water suppliers to cholera-affected areas during the epidemic were the Southwark and Vauxhall (S&V) Company and the Lambeth
Company. In 1852, the Lambeth Company moved its water collection
upstream to an area outside London and free from London's sewage,
while the S&V Company continued to draw water from a downstream
source within London. A new cholera epidemic began in 1853 and Table 1.2
shows the number of cholera deaths per 10,000 households during the
first 7 weeks of the epidemic, stratified by water supply.

Table 1.2 Water sources and cholera mortality in London, 9 July to 26 August 1854

Source of water	Total number of houses	Number of cholera deaths	Cholera deaths per 10,000 houses
S&V Company	40,046	1263	315
Lambeth Company	26,107	98	38
Rest of London	256,423	1422	55

Source: Adapted from Snow (1936).

1. Describe the data presented and compare the cholera deaths between the two water companies.
2. Do these data support Snow's hypothesis that cholera is transmitted through water? Can we conclude that the water from the S&V Company is the cause of the cholera outbreak? Give reasons for your answer.

Analytical studies

Analytical studies aim to compare the frequency of the outcome in groups or individuals with and without the exposure of interest (as done by Ramazzini, Louis, and Snow). There are four different types of analytical study:

1. **Ecological studies** consider population-level data and aim to relate the total frequency of an outcome to an average level of exposure by population group. For example, differences in alcohol consumption and incidence of breast cancer by country.
2. **Cross-sectional studies** collect data on outcome and exposure at one point in time from a random sample of study **subjects**. For example, the presence of HIV infection in relation to prior male circumcision.
3. **Cohort studies** record differences in exposure to a risk factor and follow up these individuals to measure the occurrence over time of the outcome in relation to this exposure. For example, occurrence of cervical cancer in relation to human papillomavirus infection.
4. **Case-control studies** identify individuals with the outcome (called 'cases') and without the outcome (called 'controls') and examine whether they differ in relation to previous exposure to a risk factor. For example, mobile telephone use among people with brain tumours compared with that of people without brain tumours.

Figure 1.4 shows an example of the timing of different study designs in relation to when exposure and outcome occur. A cross-sectional study

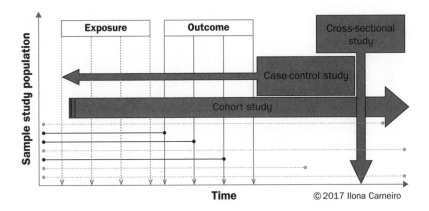

Figure 1.4 Timing of study designs in relation to exposure and outcome

Note: Solid horizontal lines represent subjects who acquire the outcome; dashed horizontal lines represent those who never acquire the outcome, but may leave the study before the end.

occurs at one point in time for a study **population** and the exposure and outcome may already have occurred for some individuals, but not for others. Consider that the cross-sectional study's arrow could be moved left or right to occur at any point along the timeline. A cohort study may start before or after some individuals have been **exposed**, and exposure could be repetitive or even cumulative. Some individuals could die of other causes or leave the study population, and the study could also finish before some individuals demonstrate the outcome (i.e. the cohort study's arrow could be shorter or longer than represented in the figure). A case-control study is conducted only after the outcome has occurred in some individuals (cases) and looks retrospectively to ascertain what proportion of the cases and controls have been exposed to a risk factor. The case-control study's arrow could be shorter or longer, as recruitment of cases and controls can be prospective, even though ascertainment of exposure is retrospective.

Intervention studies

An **intervention study** is considered the ideal epidemiological study design, as the investigators 'intervene' to allocate an exposure to individuals being studied. It is an experiment to evaluate the effect of reducing a risk factor or increasing a protective factor on the frequency of an outcome (as done by Lind in the scurvy experiment). The intervention is allocated to individuals or groups, and the frequency of the outcome in those exposed is compared with its frequency in those unexposed. For example, the incidence of malaria among children using an insecticide-treated mosquito net can be compared with the incidence among those using an untreated mosquito net. Intervention studies may be randomized or non-randomized.

✎ **Activity 1.4**

John Snow investigated one of the worst cholera outbreaks in London in August/September 1854. He produced a map of cholera deaths and identified a single water pump as the main source of the cholera. He persuaded the local authorities to remove the pump-handle on 8 September, preventing further use of the pump. Figure 1.5 shows the date of onset of symptoms for 616 fatal cases of cholera near the pump.

1. Describe what the graph in Figure 1.5 shows.
2. Did removal of the pump-handle on 8 September end the cholera outbreak? Explain your answer.

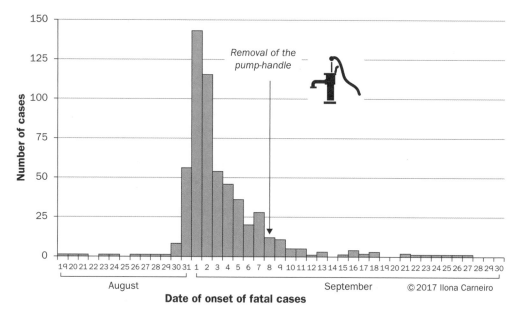

Figure 1.5 Distribution of cases of cholera by date of onset
Source: Data from Snow (1936).

Alternative reasons for association

Analytical methods may confirm an association between an exposure and outcome, but we can infer causality only if alternative explanations such as chance, bias, and confounding have been accounted for. **Chance** refers to a random result, known as **random error**, such as when a coin is tossed 10 times and lands face-up seven times. **Bias** refers to **systematic** errors that may misrepresent the association being investigated, such as if a coin had been altered so that it always landed face-up. **Confounding** is caused when another factor, independently associated with both the outcome and exposure of interest, influences the association being investigated. For example, in Farr's study of the cholera outbreaks, elevation was a confounder in the association between contaminated water and cholera. These alternative explanations for an apparent association between an outcome and an exposure, and the challenges for inferring causality, will be discussed in more detail in Chapter 4.

The application of epidemiology

Epidemiology provides scientific evidence for public health policy decisions. The data and relationships identified through epidemiological study may be used in various ways. Descriptive epidemiological methods enable health professionals to identify the actual and potential health problems in a population. The burden of health outcomes or associated risk factors can be quantified, related to existing health services, and tracked to predict changes over time. An overview of the health issues affecting a population, and more importantly the relative distribution of these health issues, enables priorities to be set and programmes to be planned.

Once a risk factor has been identified through one or more analytical studies, health promotion activities may be developed to reduce exposure to the outcome at the individual level (e.g. encouraging smokers to stop smoking through education and support programmes) or population level (e.g. banning smoking in public places). Screening programmes may be implemented to increase early diagnosis and appropriate treatment (e.g. recommending mammograms for all women over 50 years of age, who are at greater risk of breast cancer than younger women).

Monitoring and evaluation of health programmes are necessary to assess whether an implemented intervention is safe and effective under routine conditions, and whether this can be maintained over time. This may take the form of routine surveillance for the outcome (e.g. number of measles cases) or recording programmatic indicators (e.g. number of children receiving three doses of measles vaccine). These topics will be covered in more detail in Chapters 11 and 12.

Conclusion

Epidemiology includes both a scientific approach (evidenced-based medicine) and a societal perspective (population-based studies and solutions) to health. In this chapter, you have been introduced to several new concepts and terms that are key to the understanding of epidemiology (i.e. descriptive epidemiology, inferring causality, analytical study designs, interpretation of results, and the applications of epidemiology). These issues are fundamental for those involved in clinical and public health and will be discussed in more depth in subsequent chapters.

Feedback on activities in Chapter 1

Feedback on Activity 1.1

You may have written some of the following:

There were similar numbers of subjects in each group. The duration of illness was 3 days shorter in those who were first bled earlier, but their mortality was much higher ($18/41 = 44\%$ compared with $9/36 = 25\%$).

This suggests that while early bloodletting reduces the duration of pneumonia, the increased mortality rate questions the safety of this practice. Louis concluded that the beneficial effect of bloodletting was 'much less than has been commonly believed', and suggested limiting its use to severe cases.

Feedback on Activity 1.2

Your answers should include the main pattern shown and potential reasons:

1. The graph shows that the number of maternal deaths per 100,000 live births per year for the USA was highest (approximately 850/100,000 live births) in 1900 and declined rapidly between 1930 and 1950 (to approximately 100/100,000 live births) with a more gradual decline to very low levels by the end of the twentieth century.
2. This may have been due to improved obstetric practices or hygiene or any other reasonable explanation. [Additional contextual information: At the start of the twentieth century, delivery practices in the USA were poor and excessive interventions (e.g. induction of labour, use of forceps) were often performed without aseptic conditions. An increase in safer hospital deliveries under aseptic conditions between 1930 and 1950, and legalization of abortions after the 1960s, led to a decline in maternal mortality (Centers for Disease Control and Prevention, 1999).]

Feedback on Activity 1.3

1. Table 1.2 shows the number of houses receiving water from each water company compared with the rest of London. It also shows the number

of deaths from cholera per 10,000 houses (calculated by dividing the second column by the first column and multiplying by 10,000). The risk of death due to cholera was 315/10,000 in houses supplied by the S&V Company, 38/10,000 in houses supplied by the Lambeth Company, and 55/10,000 in the rest of London. These data suggest that the risk of cholera death was eight to nine times higher (315/38) in houses supplied by the S&V Company compared with the Lambeth Company.

2. These data support Snow's hypothesis that cholera is transmitted through water, but they do not prove it. We should consider the number of people per house, their socio-economic status, and other potential factors that may be associated with cholera. For example, the S&V Company may have supplied water to multiple-occupancy buildings while Lambeth supplied individual family houses. If this were the case, then the risk of cholera death per house between the two populations would not be comparable, since the average number of people per house would be different. Since the S&V Company was drawing water from downstream, it is possible that households supplied by the company would have been in downstream areas and might be poorer than households upstream. Such differences in socio-economic status may also be responsible for the increased spread of cholera or likelihood of dying from it. Although these data appear to support Snow's hypothesis, more information is needed to be sure.

Feedback on Activity 1.4

1. Figure 1.5 shows an outbreak of cholera in this population. There appears to have been a low number of cases (zero or one case per day) before 30 August. There was an explosive rise in the number of cases over 3 days, peaking at nearly 150 cases per day on 1 September. The number of cases returned to previous low levels after about 2 weeks.

2. While the timing of the reduction in cases coincides with the public health intervention (i.e. removal of the pump-handle), the number of cholera deaths had already decreased considerably before this happened. This suggests that removal of the pump-handle was not responsible for the end of the outbreak. Snow suggested two alternative explanations for the end of the outbreak: (i) many people who lived in the area moved elsewhere due to fear of contracting cholera, and (ii) the amount of causal agent in the water might somehow have been reduced. A third possibility is that **susceptible** people (i.e. those who had no form of immunity to cholera and were therefore at risk of infection) might have been infected early on, leaving few susceptible individuals to be infected later.

2 | Measuring outcome frequency

Overview

To study the distribution of a health outcome it is necessary to quantify its frequency, which is the number of occurrences in a defined population over a defined period. In this chapter, you will be introduced to the key descriptive epidemiological measures used to determine the frequency of outcomes: prevalence, risk (including attack rate), odds, and incidence rate. These are used to describe the distribution of an outcome in a population and to see how it may vary geographically, over time or between populations.

Learning objectives

When you have completed this chapter, you should be able to:

- identify and distinguish between measures of frequency – prevalence, risk, odds, and incidence rate
- define and calculate each of these frequency measures from relevant data
- recognize the use of secondary attack rates in the investigation of outbreaks
- estimate person-time at risk

Defining a case

To measure the **frequency** of an outcome, it is necessary to have a clear definition or description that identifies the outcome of interest. In some circumstances, the outcome is obvious (e.g. all-cause death), but standardized criteria are often needed (e.g. severe anaemia may be defined as haemoglobin less than 5 grams per decilitre). Individuals with the outcome of interest are often referred to as 'cases'. The criteria used to define them form the **case definition**, which may not necessarily be clinically defined. The outcome may refer to an event such as a car accident rather than an illness. A 'case' may occur only once per individual (e.g. death), more than once (e.g. pregnancy) or frequently (e.g. diarrhoeal disease). Epidemiologists count cases using clinical assessments, diagnostic tests, registry or facility record entries, observation, or even self-reporting in population surveys.

Knowing the number of cases is not enough to allow any comparison or association to be made. If you were told that there were 75 cases of tuberculosis in village A and only 25 cases in village B, you might be tempted to conclude that tuberculosis was more common in village A than in village B. However, without knowing how many people live in each village, this comparison is impossible to make. To calculate frequency, it is necessary to enumerate the population at risk.

Defining a population

The occurrence of health outcomes (e.g. infection, illness, disability, death) will vary between populations, geographical areas, and over time. In epidemiology, we study health at the population level. However, it is important to understand who is included in this 'population'. We often refer to a **target population** whose health we are investigating or whose health we wish to improve (e.g. the population of London). As it is difficult to obtain data on every individual in the target population, epidemiological studies identify a **study population** of individuals with specific relevant characteristics (e.g. people aged 18–60 living in Central London). If the study population is very large, a **sample** of individuals may be selected (usually randomly) from the study population, and this is known as the **study sample**.

The frequency of a health outcome is a measure of the number of times it occurs in a defined population during a defined period. To calculate this frequency, we need to define the **population at risk** as only those individuals who *could* develop the outcome. For example, if the outcome is pregnancy, the population at risk would include only women of child-bearing age and would exclude all men, as they are not 'at risk' of becoming pregnant! In some cases, it is not possible to know who is at risk (e.g. who does not have immunity) and so the whole population is used as an estimate.

Measuring outcome frequency

The frequency of an outcome is usually measured as the prevalence or the incidence. **Prevalence** measures the number of existing cases in a population at a defined time point, whereas **incidence** measures the number of new cases in a population over a defined period. Figure 2.1 shows liquid passing through a flask as a simplified representation of the difference between prevalence and incidence. Prevalence is concerned only with the liquid inside the flask at any given time. Incidence considers the flow of liquid into the flask.

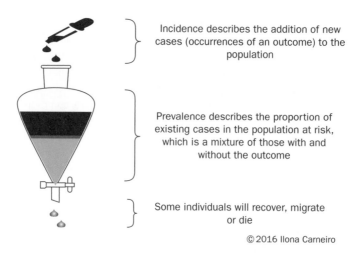

Incidence describes the addition of new cases (occurrences of an outcome) to the population

Prevalence describes the proportion of existing cases in the population at risk, which is a mixture of those with and without the outcome

Some individuals will recover, migrate or die

© 2016 Ilona Carneiro

Figure 2.1 Representation of the difference between prevalence and incidence

---

✐ Activity 2.1

Investigators were asked to determine the frequency of malaria in a village of 1000 people in rural Southeast Asia. Investigators spent a couple of days in the village testing 500 residents for malaria. Using a rapid diagnostic test (RDT) that detected malaria parasite-specific proteins in the blood, 100 people tested positive for malaria. Everybody in the village was treated with antimalarial drugs to clear any infections. Over the next 6 months, all those visiting the village health centre (accessible by all) were tested by RDT and 50 individuals tested positive for malaria.

1. Write a case definition that the investigators could have used in this study.
2. Define the study population and the study sample.
3. Based on your definitions above, how would you estimate prevalence and incidence using the data available?

Prevalence

Prevalence is defined as the number of existing cases in a population at one defined point in time divided by the total number of people at risk in that population at the same point in time. If data on the population at risk are not available, the total study population or sample population may be used as an approximation. Prevalence is calculated as:

$$\text{Prevalence} = \frac{\text{Number of existing cases}}{\text{Total population at risk at a defined point in time}}$$

Prevalence is a proportion and can never be greater than one, although it is usually presented as a percentage by multiplying the proportion by 100. It is dimensionless, meaning that it has no units, so the term 'prevalence rate' is incorrect. Prevalence is sometimes referred to as **point prevalence** to distinguish it from **period prevalence**, which refers to prevalence measured over a short period such as weeks or months.

The prevalence of an outcome may be measured during a descriptive population survey or analytical cross-sectional study. For example, in a survey of 200 boys aged 5–10 years in a low-income setting, 60 were found to be stunted (i.e. had a lower than average height-for-age), an indicator of chronic malnutrition. The prevalence of stunting in this group would be calculated as $60 \div 200 = 0.30$, which would be presented as $0.3 \times 100 = 30\%$ of young boys in this population being stunted at the time of the survey.

The number of cases present in a population at any one point depends on the frequency with which the outcome occurs ('incidence') and the duration of the outcome. If an outcome does not last long, it may be difficult to identify risk factors and to measure its impact on a population by looking at a single point in time. For example, the occurrence of an outcome with very high mortality would not be accurately measured by prevalence. If the duration of outcome varies between populations, it may also make it difficult to compare the burden. Prevalence is useful for studying the burden of chronic diseases, or for initial rapid assessment of an outcome to identify implications for health services.

Incidence

A better measure of frequency for studying causation is incidence, which is the frequency of new ('incident') cases in a defined population during a specified time. Incidence can be presented as a risk, odds or incidence **rate**, depending on how the probability of an outcome occurring is calculated. As an analogy, imagine a children's game of musical chairs, where everybody dances while the music is played and must sit on a chair when the music stops. Chairs are removed at regular intervals so that those left without a chair when the music stops must stand to one side until the game finishes. We can explain the measures of incidence as follows, where the outcome is 'sitting on a chair':

- **Risk** counts those sitting after a specified time (e.g. 10 minutes), compared with the total participants at the start of the game.
- **Odds** counts those sitting after a specified time (e.g. 10 minutes), compared with those standing after the same time.
- **Incidence rate** counts those sitting at any point during the game and considers the total time that each person participates, allowing for children who join the game late or leave early.

Using this analogy, we can also explain prevalence as the number of children sitting on a chair at any point during the game, divided by the total number of children in the game (sitting or standing). Children who are in the room but not participating in the game are not 'at risk' and are not included in either the numerator or the denominator.

Risk

Risk is also known as **cumulative incidence** because it refers to the total number of new cases in a defined 'population at risk' during a specified period. While risk is often used interchangeably with likelihood in the English language, in epidemiology it is defined specifically as:

$$\text{Risk} = \frac{\text{Number of new cases in a specified time period}}{\text{Total population at risk at the start of that time period}}$$

This measure can be interpreted as the probability that an individual will develop an outcome during a specified period. The population at risk excludes existing ('prevalent') cases at the start of the period. Risk is also a dimensionless proportion, so it has no units and has a value between zero and one. However, its value can increase with the duration of the time under consideration, making it essential to specify the period. For example, if a group of 100 people were studied for a year, and 25 had caught at least one cold during that year, we could say that the risk of catching a cold was 25 ÷ 100 = 0.25 or 25% in that group in that year. However, the result would be interpreted differently if 100 people had been studied for 6 months and 25 had caught at least one cold during this 6-month period; it would have to be specified as a 25% risk over 6 months, as it might imply a 50% risk over 12 months if there were no seasonal effect.

A specific form of risk used in disease outbreaks is called the **secondary attack rate**. This is a misnomer, as it is a proportion and not a rate (see below), but the term is widely accepted. The secondary attack rate is the number of new cases among at-risk contacts of a primary case over a specified period. It is sometimes used to show the difference between community transmission of an infection and that in a more confined population such as a household, school or workplace. A **contact** is somebody who may have interacted with an infected individual, either through direct contact (e.g. touching) or indirect contact (e.g. coughing). Secondary attack rates are calculated as follows:

$$\text{Secondary attack rate} = \frac{\text{Number of new cases among contacts in a specified time period}}{\text{Total number of contacts at risk in that time period}}$$

This can be interpreted as the probability that a contact of a primary case will develop the outcome during the specified time. For example, if eight children developed varicella (chicken pox) in an outbreak at a school of 1000 children, then the risk of infection would be 8 ÷ 1000 = 0.8%. If five out of a total of 15 siblings of these primary cases developed varicella in the subsequent 2 weeks, we could estimate the secondary attack rate, or risk of developing varicella among household contacts, as 5 ÷ 15 = 0.33 or 33% in this 2-week period. This estimate assumes that none of the siblings had been vaccinated or had any prior immunity to varicella.

Odds

Odds is a different way of representing incidence, because it compares the probability of becoming a case to the probability of not becoming a case:

$$\text{Odds} = \frac{\text{New case}}{\text{Total at risk}} \div \frac{\text{Non-cases}}{\text{Total at risk}} = \frac{\text{Cases}}{\text{Total}} \times \frac{\text{Total}}{\text{Non-cases}} = \frac{\text{Cases}}{\text{Non-cases}}$$

As both probabilities have the same denominator, these cancel out to give a simpler calculation of the number of new cases divided by the number of non-cases (individuals who did not become cases and are therefore still at risk) after a specified time:

$$\text{Odds} = \frac{\text{Number of new cases over a specified time period}}{\text{Number still at risk at the end of that time period}}$$

Notice that adding the numerator and denominator for the odds will give the total population at risk. As the **odds** are a **ratio** of two proportions, it can take any value from zero to infinity, although it is usually expressed as a ratio of integers. For example, odds of 0.33 can be written as 1:3 (calculated from the inverse of the odds, i.e. 1 ÷ 0.33). In the previous example where 25 people in a group of 100 caught a cold during one year, the odds of catching a cold would be calculated as 25 ÷ 75 = 0.33. The odds of catching a cold would be 1 to 3, reported as 1:3, so that a person in that group would be three times more likely not to catch a cold than to catch a cold during that year.

Odds are not actually used very much in epidemiology, although clinicians may use them to explain the probability of an outcome to patients. Figure 2.2 shows the relationship between odds and risk. When an outcome is very rare, there is little difference between odds and risk and there is therefore a tendency for people to use them interchangeably. However, as an outcome becomes more common, the two measures are quite different. It is often easier to interpret risks, so if you are presented with odds they can be converted using the formula:

$$\text{Risk} = \frac{\text{Odds}}{1 + \text{Odds}}$$

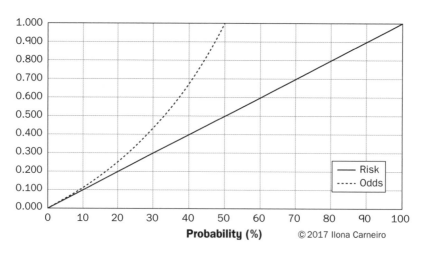

Figure 2.2 Relationship between risk and odds as the probability of an outcome increases

Incidence rate and person-time at risk

Both risk and odds assume that the population at risk is followed over a specified time, and that all those who are included at the beginning of the time are also counted at the end. This is called a 'closed' population. However, we usually want to look at incidence in a 'dynamic' or 'open' population, in which people enter and exit the population at risk at different points and are therefore at risk for different lengths of time. Once the outcome has occurred, a case will no longer be at risk or, if the outcome can recur, there will be some interval of time before that individual is once more considered at risk. Therefore, instead of counting the total number of people at the start of the study, the time is calculated that each individual is at risk. This is known as the **person-time at risk** and is illustrated in Figure 2.3. People may start and stop being at risk at different times, due to births and deaths, in or out migration, acquiring the outcome, leaving the study population before the end for unknown reasons (known as 'lost to follow-up'), or reaching the end of the observation period.

The **incidence rate** is a measure of frequency that allows us to account for variation in the time at risk. It is calculated as the number of new cases divided by the total person-time at risk:

$$\text{Incidence rate} = \frac{\text{Number of new cases in a specified time period}}{\text{Total person-time at risk during that time period}}$$

This measure is a rate and is reported as the number of new cases per person-time at risk. It is essential to specify the time units, for example person-days, person-months, person-years, or more commonly for a rare outcome 1000 person-years at risk.

✎ Activity 2.2

In Figure 2.3, the incidence rate is obtained by dividing the total number of cases by the total number of person-years at risk. Draw up a simple table to show the time at risk for each individual and calculate the incidence rate of the outcome in Figure 2.3.

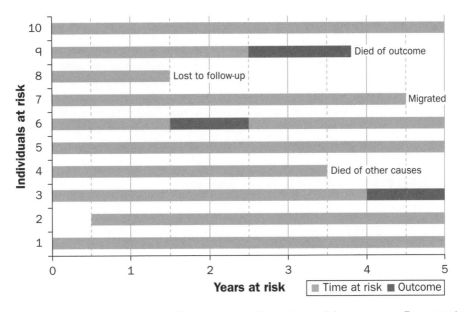

Figure 2.3 Representation of person-time at risk for 10 study participants over a 5-year period

In registry data or very large studies, it might be difficult to know the exact person-time at risk for everyone in the population. If the population size does not change substantially over the study period, we can estimate the person-time at risk from the population at risk at the period mid-point, multiplied by the total period under consideration. As an example, if we did not have information on when everyone joined and left the study in Figure 2.3, we could estimate the time at risk as the average of the population at risk that started and the population at risk that ended. As nine individuals started and five individuals were still at risk at the end, we could estimate a mid-study population at risk of $(9 + 5) \div 2 = 7$, so the total time at risk could be estimated as $7 \times 5 = 35$ person-years at risk. Cleary, this is an underestimate in this case, but when we are dealing with a very large population which is less dynamic, this estimation will better approximate the true situation.

Activity 2.3

Data from a cancer registry (a record of all cancer cases notified by doctors) found 750 cases of breast cancer in a region of a politically stable country between the beginning of 2010 and beginning of 2015. The population of that region was recorded from a census to be 100,130 in 2012. Estimate the person-time at risk and calculate the breast cancer incidence rate for this population.

Population outcomes such as births, deaths, cancer incidence, etc. are usually reported as incidence rates using an estimated mid-point population as the denominator. The calculation is often the same as for risks, although the difference is that risks use the population at the start of the period of observation as the denominator. For rare outcomes, they will often approximate to the same number, but the convention is to call them rates and to refer to person-years or 1000s or 100,000s of person-years at risk.

Relationship between prevalence and incidence

In summary, prevalence indicates how widespread an outcome is in a population and provides an estimate of the burden of that outcome for the health services. Prevalence is dependent on both the incidence and the duration of the outcome. As the incidence of an outcome increases, so too does its prevalence. In general, the prevalence will also increase as the duration of an outcome increases. The incidence indicates the risk of an outcome occurring, and does not vary with the duration of that outcome. This may result in a low incidence and high prevalence for some chronic outcomes, such as diabetes, or a high incidence and low prevalence for a short duration outcome such as the common cold.

Conclusion

You have been introduced to the important measures of prevalence and incidence that are used to quantify the occurrence of an outcome in a defined population in both descriptive and analytical studies. Prevalence tends to be used for chronic outcomes and for the rapid assessment of the burden of an outcome. Risk and incidence rate indicate the probability of an outcome occurring, and are more useful for studying its causes. Odds are rarely used in epidemiology. Incidence rates are also used to describe the occurrence of population-level outcomes such as births and deaths (mortality rate). These epidemiological measures of frequency help to assess the public health importance of an outcome and to plan appropriate health service responses. They also form the basis of analytical studies to investigate the association between exposures and outcomes, as you will learn in Chapter 3.

Additional activities to test your understanding

✎ Activity 2.4

For each of the following examples, identify whether the measure of frequency is a prevalence, risk or incidence rate, and give reasons for your answer:

1. $$\frac{\text{Number of women diagnosed with breast cancer in study A}}{\text{Number of women initially enrolled in study A}}$$

2. $$\frac{\text{Number newly diagnosed with tuberculosis in study Y between 2005 and 2010}}{\text{Number of person-years at risk in Study Y during the same period}}$$

3. $$\frac{\text{Number of children with asthma in School X on the first day of term}}{\text{Number of children enrolled in School X on the first day of term}}$$

4. $$\frac{\text{Number of road traffic deaths in City B in 2015}}{\text{Estimated number of people living in City B on 30 June 2015}}$$

✎ Activity 2.5

Investigators conducted a survey of intestinal worm infestation among 1000 adolescent agricultural workers in Country Y. They found 620 adolescents were infested with one or more types of worm. After treating all adolescents found positive, investigators returned 6 months later and tested all 1000 adolescents again. This time they found 330 adolescents infested.

1. Calculate the prevalence of worm infestation among adolescents in the first survey.

2. Calculate the risk and the odds of worm infestation among adolescents during the 6-month study period.
3. What is the incidence rate of worm infestation among adolescents during the 6-month study period?

✐ Activity 2.6

An outbreak of human monkeypox, a relatively rare orthopox viral disease related to smallpox, was detected in the Democratic Republic of Congo (DRC). Investigators found five secondary cases of monkeypox among 37 household contacts of a 9-year-old boy who was the first reported to have become infected.

1. Assuming all household contacts are equally at risk, what is the secondary attack rate among household contacts?
2. Data from previous outbreaks suggests that prior smallpox vaccination confers some protection from monkeypox. Estimate a new secondary attack rate if 27 household contacts had been vaccinated against smallpox.

Feedback on activities in Chapter 2

Feedback on Activity 2.1

1. Cases could be defined as those individuals who were resident in the village and tested positive for malaria by rapid diagnostic test.
2. The study population includes all 1000 individuals in the study village. The study sample for the survey was the subset of 500 people who were tested for malaria.
3. Prevalence is the proportion of existing cases in the population at risk at the time of the study. Therefore, only those 500 who were tested could have been 'at risk' of testing positive for malaria, and 100 did test positive, so the prevalence of existing malaria would be the proportion positive: 100 ÷ 500 = 1/5, or 0.20 or 20%.

   Incidence can be calculated from the number of new cases in the population during the 6 months of testing at the health centre. Assuming all members of the village could have attended the health centre, the population at risk would now be 1000. The number of new cases was

50, so the incidence would be the proportion of new cases: 50 ÷ 1000 = 5/100, or 0.05 or 5% over the 6-month observation period.

You may have given slightly different answers to those above. This activity was intended to get you to question how outcome frequency is measured, and any doubts you may have should be clarified as you work through the rest of the chapter.

Feedback on Activity 2.2

Table 2.1 shows the time at risk for each individual.

Table 2.1 Tabulation of person-time at risk in Figure 2.3

Individual	Time at risk	Comments
1	5.0	Full 5-years at risk
2	4.5	Became at risk after 0.5 years
3	4.0	Outcome at 4 years until end of study
4	3.5	Died at 3.5 years of other causes
5	5.0	Full 5-years at risk
6	4.0	Outcome from 1.5 to 2.5 years, then recovered and was again at risk until study end
7	4.5	At risk until leaving the study at 4.5 years
8	1.5	Left study at 1.5 years – unknown reason
9	2.5	Outcome at 2.5 years, then died of outcome
10	5.0	Full 5-years at risk
Total	39.5	

Three individuals (numbers 3, 6, and 9) became cases during the 5-year period. A total of 39.5 person-years at risk were observed during the study. The incidence of this outcome was 3 ÷ 39.5 = 0.076 cases per person-year at risk, or 76 cases per 1000 person-years at risk (when we convert it to whole numbers to make it clearer).

Feedback on Activity 2.3

The person-time at risk is estimated as the mid-period population from the census in 2012 multiplied by the 5-year period at risk: $100,130 \times 5 = 500,650$ person-years at risk. The incidence is calculated as 750 ÷ 500,650 = 0.0015 per person-year at risk, or 1.5 cases of breast cancer per 1000 person-years at risk between 2010 and 2014.

Feedback on Activity 2.4

1. Risk, because the numerator is the number of new cases and the denominator is the population at risk at the start of the study period.
2. Incidence rate, because the numerator is the number of new cases and the denominator is the person-time at risk for the same period.
3. Prevalence, because the numerator is the number of existing cases of asthma at one time point and the denominator is the total number at risk at the same time point.
4. Incidence rate, because the numerator is the number of 'new cases' during the year and the denominator is the mid-year population. You may have said risk because there is no reference to time at risk, but it is not the population at the start of the period at risk.

Feedback on Activity 2.5

1. The number of existing cases of worm infestation in the first survey = 620. The total number of adolescents tested was 1000. Therefore, the prevalence of infestation among adolescents in the first survey was $(620 \div 1000) \times 100 = 0.62 \times 100 = 62\%$.
2. The number of incident cases of worm infestation in the second survey = 330. The total number of adolescents at risk was 1000. Therefore, the risk of infestation among adolescents during the 6-month period was $(330 \div 1000) \times 100 = 0.33 \times 100 = 33\%$.

    Note that if there were no pre-existing cases (e.g. because all cases had been successfully treated), then the new prevalence at the end of the study period is equivalent to the risk.

    The number of cases in the second survey = 330. The number of adolescents who were not cases (still at risk) = 1000 − 330 = 670. Therefore, the odds of infestation among adolescents during the 6-month period were $(330 \div 670) = 0.49$ or 1:2.
3. The number of incident cases in the second survey = 330. We do not know when each person became infested or how many months each adolescent was at risk. Therefore, we need to calculate the mid-period population as the average of the population at the start and end of the study. At the end, there were only 670 adolescents still at risk, so the mid-period population was (1000 + 670)/2 = 835. The study period was 6 months, so the time at risk was 835 × 6 = 5010 person-months, assuming that adolescents did not leave the study area for significant periods during that time period. Therefore, the incidence rate of infestation among these adolescents is estimated as $(330 \div 5010) = 0.066 \times 1000 = 66$. Therefore, the incidence rate when rounded up was 66 infestations per 1000 person-months.

Feedback on Activity 2.6

1. The number of cases of monkeypox among secondary contacts = 5. The total number of secondary household contacts = 37. Therefore, the secondary attack rate = $5 \div 37 \times 100 = 0.135 \times 100 = 13.5\%$.
2. If 27 contacts had been vaccinated against smallpox, then $37 - 27 = 10$ household contacts were unprotected. The number of cases of monkeypox among household contacts was 5. Therefore, the secondary attack rate would be $5 \div 10 = 50\%$. This would indicate that monkeypox was much more virulent than originally estimated.

3 Measuring association and effect

Overview

In analytical epidemiology, the aim is to quantify the association between an exposure and an outcome to detect causal relationships that may help identify effective interventions. We use the measures of frequency from the previous chapter to compare outcomes in different exposure groups using four relative frequency comparisons: prevalence ratio, risk ratio, odds ratio, and incidence rate ratio.

If there is evidence of a causal association, we can assess the impact of an exposure as an absolute difference in frequency between the exposure groups using attributable risk, attributable fraction, and preventable fraction. To estimate the public health impact of removing an exposure, we calculate the population attributable fraction.

Learning objectives

When you have completed this chapter, you should be able to:

- identify different measures of association – prevalence ratio, risk ratio, odds ratio, and incidence rate ratio
- recognize different measures of impact – attributable risk, attributable fraction, preventable fraction, and population attributable fraction
- define, calculate, and interpret each measure of association and impact
- use an appropriate measure of association or impact for a given objective

Measures of association

To estimate the strength or amount of an association between an exposure and an outcome, we use relative measures to compare the frequency of an outcome between two or more exposure groups. These measures of prevalence ratio, risk ratio, odds ratio, and incidence rate ratio are collectively referred to as measures of **relative risk**. However, it is good practice to refer to specific relative risk measures by name, to avoid confusing the term 'relative risk' with the specific 'risk ratio' measure.

In Chapter 1, we saw how John Snow compared the risk of cholera deaths in households served by different water companies and found an eight- to nine-fold difference in deaths between them. We don't often see such stark effects, and therefore need to decide what magnitude of association is of public health importance. The issues to consider include: the severity of the outcome and its implications, the economic costs of the outcome to the individual and to society, and the costs of prevention or intervention.

To calculate a measure of association, we usually nominate one group as 'exposed' to an outcome of interest and the comparison group as 'unexposed'. A relative risk divides the frequency of outcome in those exposed by that in the unexposed, to indicate how much more likely the outcome is to occur with the exposure. As relative risks are ratios, they can take any value between zero and infinity. If the relative risk is greater than one (RR > 1), exposed individuals are at greater risk. If the relative risk equals one (RR = 1), there is no difference in risk between the exposed and unexposed groups. And if the relative risk is less than one (RR < 1), exposed individuals are at a lower risk, and the exposure can be called a protective factor. The further away the RR is from 1, the stronger the measured association.

Figure 3.1 shows how the value of a relative risk relates to the magnitude of increase or decrease in an outcome, using the relationship (RR – 1) × 100. For example, if the relative risk is 0.5, then this equates to half the frequency, or (0.5 – 1) × 100 = –50%, which is a 50% reduction in the outcome in the exposed group. If the relative risk is 3, then this equates to a three times greater frequency, or (3 – 1) × 100 = 200%, which is a 200% increase in the outcome in the exposed group.

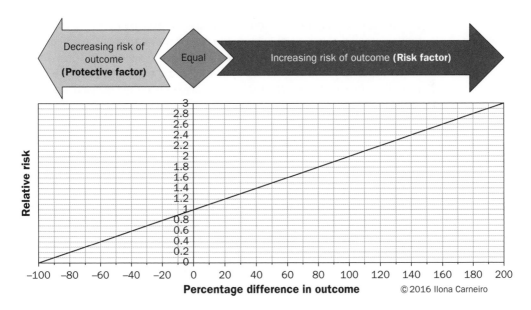

Figure 3.1 The conversion of relative risk to percentage increase or decrease in outcome

Table 3.1 Standard cross-tabulation (2 × 2 table) of outcome by exposure

	Outcome		
Exposure	Yes	No	*Total*
Yes	*a*	*b*	*a + b*
No	*c*	*d*	*c + d*
Total	*a + c*	*b + d*	*a + b + c + d*

Table 3.1 illustrates the standard format for presenting comparative data in an epidemiological study and will be used to clarify the differences between the different measures of relative risk.

Prevalence ratio

The **prevalence ratio** can be calculated from cross-sectional studies or population surveys that measure the prevalence of an outcome. It is calculated as the prevalence in exposed individuals divided by the prevalence in unexposed individuals:

$$\text{Prevalence ratio} = \frac{\text{Prevalence of outcome in exposed group}}{\text{Prevalence of outcome in unexposed group}}$$

If Table 3.1 is taken to represent the number of existing cases by exposure group detected at one point in time, the overall prevalence of the outcome in the sample population is calculated as $(a + c)/(a + b + c + d)$. The prevalence in the exposed group is given by $a/(a + b)$ and the prevalence in the unexposed group is given by $c/(c + d)$, so the prevalence ratio is calculated as:

$$\text{Prevalence ratio} = \frac{a/(a + b)}{c/(c + d)}$$

It is not necessary to know the actual number of cases or the total number of individuals, if the prevalence in each exposure group is known. For example, you are told that the prevalence of obesity, defined as body mass index greater than 30 kg/m², is 20% in people who report that they do less than 2 hours of exercise per week, and 10% in those who report that they do at least 2 hours of exercise per week. The prevalence ratio for obesity can be calculated as $0.10 \div 0.20 = 0.50$ in those 'exposed' to at least 2 hours of exercise per week. This measure of association between the prevalence of obesity and exercise can be interpreted as exposed individuals (i.e. those who exercise for at least 2 hours per week) being 0.50 times or half as likely to be obese as unexposed individuals (i.e. those who did not exercise for at least 2 hours per week). The ratio can also be inverted as $0.20 \div 0.10 = 2.0$, such that those who did less than 2 hours of exercise per week are twice as likely to be obese as those who did at least 2 hours of exercise per week.

Risk ratio

The **risk ratio** can be calculated from ecological or cohort studies. The risk ratio is calculated as the risk (cumulative incidence) of the outcome in the exposed group divided by the risk (cumulative incidence) of the outcome in the unexposed group:

$$\text{Risk ratio} = \frac{\text{Risk of outcome in exposed group}}{\text{Risk of outcome in unexposed group}}$$

If Table 3.1 is taken to represent the number of new (incident) cases by exposure group detected during a defined period of time, the overall risk of the outcome in the sample population can be calculated as $(a + c)/(a + b + c + d)$. The risk in the exposed group is given by $a/(a + b)$ and the risk in the unexposed group is given by $c/(c + d)$, so the risk ratio can be calculated as:

$$\text{Risk ratio} = \frac{a/(a + b)}{c/(c + d)}$$

Note that these equations are identical to those for prevalence, because risk is also a proportion as discussed in the previous chapter, but can only be applied to incident cases. For example, a cohort study observed that 20 out of 50 children who regularly washed their hands with soap after defecation had at least one episode of diarrhoea during the study period, compared with 20 out of 40 children who did not. The risk ratio can be calculated as $(20 \div 50)/(20 \div 40) = 0.4 \div 0.5 = 0.80$. This is interpreted as children who practise hand washing with soap (exposed) being 0.8 times as likely, or 20% less likely (see Figure 3.1), to have diarrhoea than those who do not wash their hands with soap (unexposed).

Odds ratio

The **odds ratio of outcome** is not often calculated in epidemiological studies, but is often the result of logistic regression analyses (see Chapter 5). It is calculated as the odds of the outcome in the exposed group divided by the odds of the outcome in the unexposed group:

$$\text{Odds ratio of outcome} = \frac{\text{Odds of outcome in exposed group}}{\text{Odds of outcome in unexposed group}}$$

Referring to Table 3.1, the odds of cases in the total population are calculated as $(a + c)/(b + d)$. Reading across the table, the odds in the exposed group are a/b and the odds in the unexposed group are c/d, so the odds ratio of outcome can be calculated as follows:

$$\text{Odds ratio of outcome} = \frac{a/b}{c/d}$$

When a fraction is divided by a fraction, it can be simplified by multiplying the top and bottom of the equation by the denominators b and d:

$$\text{Odds ratio of outcome} = \frac{a/b}{c/d} \times \frac{b \times d}{b \times d} = \frac{ad}{bc}$$

A more commonly used version is the **odds ratio of exposure**, which is the *only* appropriate measure of association in case-control studies. Case-control studies focus on those with the outcome of interest and a selected comparison group without the outcome (see Chapter 9). Individuals are selected based on their outcome status (cases or controls), thus the frequency of the outcome in the population cannot be measured since we don't have a random sample of the population at risk. However, the frequency of exposure can be compared between the two outcome groups. This is calculated as the odds of exposure in individuals with the outcome (cases) divided by the odds of exposure in individuals without the outcome (controls):

$$\text{Odds ratio of exposure} = \frac{\text{Odds of exposure in those with the outcome}}{\text{Odds of exposure in those without the outcome}}$$

Referring to Table 3.1 and reading downwards, the odds of exposure in those with the outcome is a/c, and the odds of exposure in those without the outcome is b/d, so the odds ratio of exposure is:

$$\text{Odds ratio of exposure} = \frac{a/c}{b/d} = \frac{a/c}{b/d} \times \frac{c \times d}{c \times d} = \frac{ad}{bc}$$

As you can see, the odds ratio of exposure is mathematically the same as the odds ratio of outcome given above. However, it is important not to use the two terms interchangeably, as they are conceptually very different. We cannot calculate the odds ratio of outcome from a case-control study because we do not know the true odds or probability of the outcome in the study population, having specifically identified individuals based on their outcome. Try the following activity to see how these two measures compare.

✎ **Activity 3.1**

---

1. One thousand mothers of newborn babies in a low-income Sub-Saharan African country were asked about their level of education: 400 had completed primary education, while 600 had not. After one year, 16 infants 'exposed' to mothers who had completed primary education had died and 48 'unexposed' infants had died. Draw up a 2 × 2 table of these results, calculate the odds ratio of outcome, and interpret your result.

2. In a case-control study in the same country, 100 infant deaths were identified among hospital admissions, and 100 infants who survived were selected for comparison from admissions to the same hospital. In a questionnaire conducted at admission, 20 of the mothers of infants who subsequently died reported that they had completed primary education, compared with 35 of the mothers of infants who survived. Draw up a 2 × 2 table of these results, calculate the odds ratio of exposure, and interpret your result.

3. Compare your findings from questions (1) and (2) above, and explain the difference in interpretation between the two measures you calculated.

Incidence rate ratio

The **incidence rate ratio** can be obtained from ecological or cohort studies. It is calculated as the incidence rate of the outcome in the exposed group divided by the incidence rate of the outcome in the unexposed group:

$$\text{Incidence rate ratio} = \frac{\text{Incidence rate of outcome in the exposed group}}{\text{Incidence rate of outcome in the unexposed group}}$$

Referring again to Table 3.1, the column for 'no outcome' would in this instance be replaced by the person-time at risk. The incidence rate of the outcome in the total sample population can then be calculated as $(a + c)/(b + d)$. The incidence rate in the exposed group is a/b and the incidence rate in the unexposed group is c/d. As with the odds ratio, the incidence rate ratio can be simplified as follows:

$$\text{Incidence rate ratio} = \frac{a/b}{c/d} = \frac{ad}{bc}$$

We use the incidence rate ratio when our measure of frequency is the incidence rate. This is usually in dynamic studies where people are entering and leaving the study population or have varying levels of exposure. It is also traditionally used for large population-based or routinely collected data such as mortality rates or cancer incidence (although these could be reported as risks if the person-time at risk is the same for all exposure groups).

✎ **Activity 3.2**

A cohort study had the aim of measuring the association between hypertension and type 2 diabetes incidence in 1100 men who were followed up over 7 years. Of those without hypertension at enrolment, 54 were diagnosed with diabetes during 11,235 person-years of follow-up. Of those with hypertension, 36 were diagnosed with diabetes during 3500 person-years of follow-up.

1. Draw up a 2 × 2 table to present these data.
2. Calculate the incidence rate in the exposed and unexposed groups.
3. Calculate the incidence rate ratio to show the association between hypertension and type 2 diabetes, and interpret your result.

Comparability of measures of association

For common outcomes, such as many infectious diseases, the measures of association above may differ substantially. For rare outcomes, such as most cancers, congenital malformations, and deaths, the risk ratio and odds ratio may be very similar. To demonstrate this, consider the data in Table 3.2 for an outcome with a population incidence risk of $15 \div 10{,}000 = 0.15\%$:

- Risk ratio = $(10 \div 5000)/(5 \div 5000) = 0.002 \div 0.001 = 2.00$
- Odds ratio of outcome = $(10 \div 4990)/(5 \div 4995) = 0.002 \div 0.001 = 2.00$

Table 3.2 Table of outcome versus exposure from a hypothetical Study A

	Outcome		
Exposure	Yes	No	*Total*
Yes	10	4990	5000
No	5	4995	5000
Total	15	9985	10,000

The rarer the outcome, the more the denominator for the odds resembles the denominator for the risk (i.e. the total population at risk), and the more similar are the measures of association. This relationship is also dependent on the frequency of the exposure, making it difficult to define a threshold for this 'rare disease' assumption. If the exposure is more common, then the measures of association will also tend to be more similar. The following activity gives you an opportunity to practise these concepts.

✎ Activity 3.3

1. For the data in Table 3.3, calculate the population risk of outcome, population risk of exposure, risk ratio, and odds ratio for Study B. Compare your findings with the example given in the text above for Study A.

Table 3.3 Data from a hypothetical Study B

	Outcome		
Exposure	Yes	No	Total
Yes	10	90	100
No	5	95	100
Total	15	185	200

2. For the data in Table 3.4, calculate the population risk of outcome, population risk of exposure, risk ratio, and odds ratio for Study C. Compare your findings with the example given in question (1) for Study B.

Table 3.4 Data from a hypothetical Study C

	Outcome		
Exposure	Yes	No	Total
Yes	6	44	50
No	9	141	150
Total	15	185	200

You will often see the odds ratio (of outcome) presented in a study that has measured prevalence or risk. It is used to approximate the prevalence ratio or risk ratio when logistic regression – a type of statistical modelling – is used for analysis (see Chapter 5). However, it is worth remembering that this approximation is valid only for rare outcomes. The odds ratio will tend to overestimate the prevalence ratio or risk ratio if the outcome is not sufficiently rare, or if the exposure is rare.

Measures of effect

The measures of association described above are relative risks that show how strongly an exposure is associated with a particular outcome, and may give an indication of causality (see Chapter 4). However, they do not tell us the importance for public health. If an outcome is very rare, we may be less concerned about an exposure associated with an increased risk than for a common outcome. For example, an exposure that doubled the risk of adult asthma might be more worrying in a country where the prevalence is estimated to be over 20%, compared with a country where the prevalence is estimated to be around 2%.

To determine how much of an outcome can be explained by (attributed to) a specific exposure, we calculate the **attributable risk** as the additional outcome that occurs in exposed individuals compared with unexposed individuals in the same population (see Figure 3.2). There is usually more than one factor responsible for an outcome in epidemiology. For example, while most lung cancer is blamed on tobacco smoke, about 25% of lung cancers worldwide occur in individuals who have never smoked. The frequency occurring in unexposed individuals is called the **background risk** of the outcome.

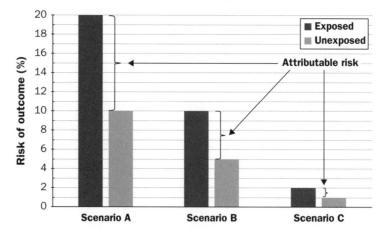

Figure 3.2 Attributable risk is the excess risk in the exposed group compared with the unexposed group

If we can assume that the exposure is causally associated with the outcome (see Chapter 4), then the attributable risk is calculated by subtracting the frequency of outcome in unexposed individuals ('background risk') from that in exposed individuals in the same population:

Attributable risk = Frequency in exposed − Frequency in unexposed

✎ Activity 3.4

Figure 3.2 shows three different scenarios where individuals are exposed or not to a hypothetical risk factor.

1. Calculate the risk ratio for each of the scenarios shown in Figure 3.2.
2. Calculate the attributable risk for each of the scenarios shown in Figure 3.2.
3. Compare your results from questions (1) and (2), and explain what different information the two measures give about the risk of outcome for an individual that is exposed to the risk factor in each of the scenarios.

Clinicians sometimes present this information as a proportion (fraction) of the outcome in exposed individuals that can be attributed to the exposure, to explain the increased risk of an exposure to a patient. This is called the **attributable fraction** and is calculated as:

$$\text{Attributable fraction} = \frac{\text{Frequency in exposed} - \text{Frequency in unexposed}}{\text{Frequency in exposed}}$$

or

$$\text{Attributable fraction} = \frac{\text{Attributable risk}}{\text{Frequency in exposed}}$$

✎ Activity 3.5

Calculate and interpret the attributable fraction for each of the scenarios shown in Figure 3.2.

You may have realized that the attributable fraction is related to the relative risk in the following way:

$$\text{Attributable fraction} = 1 - \frac{1}{\text{Relative risk}}$$

This is useful if we do not know the actual incidence of the outcome, as in case-control studies. We often use this approach to measure the effect of a **protective factor** (e.g. a genetic attribute), where the incidence among unexposed individuals is greater than the incidence among exposed individuals. This is called the **preventable fraction** and is calculated as:

$$\text{Preventable fraction} = \frac{\text{Frequency in unexposed} - \text{Frequency in exposed}}{\text{Frequency in unexposed}}$$

or

Preventable fraction = 1 − Relative risk

When calculated for an intervention (e.g. a vaccine against an infectious disease), the result is referred to as the **protective efficacy** (see Chapter 10).

Population-level measures

For public health planning, we need to apply these measures of effect to a real population. Such population measures of impact are specific to the population for which they are calculated because they vary with the frequency and distribution of the exposure in that population.

The absolute impact of a proposed intervention can be calculated from the **population attributable risk**. This is the excess outcome in the total population (i.e. exposed and unexposed to the risk factor) that can be attributed to the exposure, again assuming a causal relationship between exposure and outcome. It is calculated as:

Population attributable risk

= Frequency in population − Frequency in unexposed

A relative measure of impact is the **population attributable fraction** (PAF), which is the proportion (fraction) of the outcome that could be prevented if the exposure could be eliminated from the population. It is calculated as the excess outcome as a proportion of the frequency in the total population:

Population attributable fraction

$$= \frac{\text{Frequency in population} - \text{Frequency in unexposed}}{\text{Frequency in population}}$$

The PAF can be estimated using the relative risk from an epidemiological study, if the prevalence of exposure in the population of interest ('p') is known and the relative risk (RR) has been adjusted for confounding effects (see Chapter 4):

$$\text{Population attributable fraction} = \frac{p \times (\text{Relative risk} - 1)}{1 + p \times (\text{Relative risk} - 1)}$$

Similarly, it can be estimated from the prevalence of exposure among the cases only (p_c') after adjustment for confounding:

$$\text{Population attributable fraction} = p_c \left(\frac{RR - 1}{RR} \right)$$

Note, the population attributable fraction is rarely 100%, because an outcome is usually the result of more than one factor, and there is usually some outcome (background risk) in the unexposed group. As several risk factors for an outcome may overlap or interact (see pp. 13–15), reducing exposure to one risk factor may result in an increase in the proportion of cases due to another risk factor. This means that the PAF is often an overestimate of what we can truly achieve with an intervention. However, it is common practice to assume that risk factors do not overlap, and to estimate an additive PAF for multiple exposures.

Individual versus population perspective

The comparative value of the attributable fraction and the population attributable fraction can be illustrated by the following hypothetical example. A study determined the risk of repetitive strain injury (RSI) to the hand in office workers to be 4% over a one-year period. Among those who used a computer keyboard for more than 5 hours per day (exposed) the risk was 10%, while for those who used a computer keyboard for less than 5 hours (unexposed) the risk was 3%. The attributable fraction calculates the proportion of RSI due to keyboard use for more than 5 hours per day as $(10 - 3) \div 10 = 0.70$ or 70%. This is perhaps more meaningful than just saying that there is a relative risk of $10 \div 3 = 3.33$, i.e. more than three times greater risk of RSI in those that use the keyboard for more than 5 hours per day. The PAF calculates the proportion of RSI due to computer keyboard use for more than 5 hours a day among all the office workers as $(4 - 3) \div 4 = 0.25$ or 25%. In considering whether to invest in ergonomic keyboards, the employer may not consider a 25% increased risk in RSI overall to be of sufficient importance, whereas the individual would consider a 70% increase in their own risk of RSI to be considerable. This result could be used to advocate for a workstation assessment followed by a needs-based provision of ergonomic keyboards.

Activity 3.6

A study of the effect of chronic hepatitis B infection on liver cancer found that the incidence rate of liver cancer was 4 per 100,000 person-years in those without chronic hepatitis B infection and 94 per 100,000 person-years in the entire population. Assuming a causal relationship between hepatitis B infection and liver cancer:

1. Calculate the population attributable risk of chronic hepatitis B infection in this study and interpret its meaning.
2. Calculate the population attributable fraction of chronic hepatitis B infection in this study and interpret its meaning.

Activity 3.7

In 1951, 34,440 male British doctors responded to a questionnaire about their smoking habits. Over the following 20 years, more than 10,000 certified causes of death were recorded among these doctors (Doll and Peto, 1976). Doctors were classified by their smoking habits (e.g. never smoked, cigarette smoker, cigar, pipe). The age-adjusted annual death rates per 100,000 male doctors for lung cancer and ischaemic heart disease (IHD) among cigarette smokers and non-smokers are given in Table 3.5. [*Note*: This is a comparative table, not a 2 × 2 table of outcome by exposure. These are selected data, not data for the whole study population.]

Table 3.5 Cause of death and specific death rates by selected smoking habits of British male doctors, 1951–1971

	Annual death rate per 100,000 doctors	
Cause of death	Non-smokers	Cigarette smokers
Lung cancer	10	140
Ischaemic heart disease	413	669

Source: Selected data from Doll and Peto (1976).

1. Calculate an appropriate epidemiological measure to assess the strength of association between cigarette smoking and lung cancer deaths, and between smoking and IHD deaths.
2. Based on your calculations, mortality from which of the two diseases is most strongly associated with cigarette smoking?

3. Using the data in Table 3.5, calculate how many deaths per year from each disease can be attributed to cigarette smoking, and compare your findings with those from question (2).
4. What proportions of deaths from lung cancer and IHD among cigarette smokers are due to cigarette smoking? What assumptions do these measures involve?

Conclusion

You have been introduced to the relative measures (prevalence ratio, risk ratio, odds ratio, and incidence rate ratio) that are used to quantify the association between an exposure and an outcome. These measures are the foundation of analytical epidemiology, and you will have the opportunity to consider them in context in subsequent chapters relating to specific study designs. You have also been introduced to key measures of impact (attributable risk, preventable fraction, population attributable risk, and population attributable fraction) that are helpful in translating research findings into information of public health value.

Feedback on activities in Chapter 3

Feedback on Activity 3.1

Table 3.6 Cross-tabulation of results from question (1): incidence of infant deaths by maternal education

Exposure	Outcome		
Maternal education	Died	Survived	Total
Primary level	16	384	400
No primary level	48	552	600
Total	64	936	1000

1. Table 3.6 shows the distribution of infant deaths by maternal education. The *odds ratio of outcome* can be calculated as $(16 \div 384)/(48 \div 552) = 0.042 \div 0.087 = 0.479$. If we subtract 1 from this figure (i.e. $0.48 - 1 = -0.52$), this can be interpreted as 52% lower odds of dying in infancy among those born to mothers who had completed primary education compared with those who had not.

Table 3.7 Cross-tabulation of results from question (2): maternal education by number of cases and controls

Exposure	Outcome		
Maternal education	Died (Case)	Survived (Control)	*Total*
Primary level	20	35	55
No primary level	80	65	145
Total	100	100	200

2. Table 3.7 shows the distribution of maternal education by number of cases and controls. The *odds ratio of exposure* to maternal primary education can be calculated as $(20 \div 80)/(35 \div 65) = 0.250 \div 0.538 = 0.464$. If we subtract 1 from this (i.e. $0.46 - 1 = -0.54$), this can be interpreted as 54% lower odds of having a mother who had completed primary education among infants who died compared with those who survived. This is a measure of association between maternal education and infant mortality, but it is not the odds ratio of an infant dying because we do not know the true odds of infants dying in this population. It would therefore be incorrect to report this as 54% lower odds of dying among infants who had a mother who had completed primary education.

3. Both studies showed a similar association between maternal education and infant mortality. However, in the first study we saw 52% lower odds of an infant dying if their mother had completed primary education, while in the second study we saw that infants who died had a 54% lower odds of having a mother who had completed primary education. [Note that we would not normally calculate the odds ratio of outcome, unless the data were analysed using logistic regression (see Chapter 5).]

   The first study is a cohort study, in which women with an identified exposure status (primary education) are followed up to assess the incidence of a specific outcome (infant death). The second is a case-control study, in which infants with or without an outcome (infant death) are identified and then their mothers are asked about their education (exposure). In a cohort study, we know the exposure and wait for an outcome to occur, whereas in a case-control study, we know the outcome and look back to identify prior exposure.

Feedback on Activity 3.2

1. Table 3.8 shows a 2 × 2 table of the data reported.
2. The incidence rate of diabetes among those without hypertension was $54 \div 11,235 = 0.005$, which may be reported as 5 per 1000 person-years. The incidence rate of diabetes among those with hypertension was $36 \div 3500 = 0.010$ or 10 per 1000 person-years.

Table 3.8 Data on diabetes incident cases and person-time at risk by hypertension status at enrolment

Exposure	Outcome	
Hypertension	Type 2 diabetes	Person-years at risk
Yes	36	3500
No	54	11,235
Total	90	14,735

3. The incidence rate ratio can be calculated as 10 ÷ 5 = 2, which can be interpreted as the incidence of type 2 diabetes being twice as high among men with hypertension at the start of the study compared with men without hypertension. A more precise calculation would have avoided rounding the incidence rates and would have calculated the answer as (36/3,500) ÷ (54/11,235) = 2.14 or 2.14 times higher incidence among those with hypertension.

   Alternatively, you may have calculated the inverse as 5 ÷ 10 = 0.50 or a 50% lower incidence of Type 2 diabetes among men without hypertension. Or more precisely, (54/11,235) ÷ (36/3,500) = 0.47 or a 53% lower incidence among men without hypertension. Both answers are correct, depending on whether we want to focus on higher incidence in men with hypertension or lower incidence in men without hypertension.

Feedback on Activity 3.3

1. In Table 3.3, the population risk of outcome is 15 ÷ 200 = 0.075 or 7.5%. The population risk of exposure is 100 ÷ 200 = 0.50 or 50%. The risk ratio is (10 ÷ 100)/(5 ÷ 100) = 0.10 ÷ 0.05 = 2.00. The odds ratio is (10 ÷ 90)/(5 ÷ 95) = 0.111 ÷ 0.053 = 2.11.

   In Study A, the population risk of exposure was 5000 ÷ 10,000 = 0.50 or 50%, i.e. the same as here. The risk ratio was also 2.00, meaning the probability of having the outcome was twice as great if you had been exposed in both studies. However, the risk of outcome in the study population was much lower in this study (0.15% compared with 7.5%). Whereas the risk ratio and odds ratio were the same in Study A, they are no longer the same with a more frequent outcome in Study B.

2. In Table 3.4, the population risk of outcome is 15 ÷ 200 = 0.075 or 7.5%. The population risk of exposure is 50 ÷ 200 = 0.25 or 25%. The risk ratio is (6/50) ÷ (9/150) = 2.00. The odds ratio is (6/44) ÷ (9/141) = 2.14.

   In Study B, the population risk of outcome was the same at 7.5%; however, the probability of being exposed was 50% compared with 25%

here, i.e. the exposure is less common in Study C. The risk ratio is still 2.00 and the odds ratio is still greater (2.14) in this example, but they are now even less similar than for Study B.

Feedback on Activity 3.4

1. For Scenario A, the risk ratio = $20 \div 10 = 2$. For Scenario B, the risk ratio = $10 \div 5 = 2$. And for Scenario C, the risk ratio = $2 \div 1 = 2$.
2. For Scenario A, the attributable risk is $20 - 10 = 10$. For Scenario B, the attributable risk is $10 - 5 = 5$. And for Scenario C, the attributable risk is $2 - 1 = 1$. All results assume causality.
3. While the risk ratios are the same for all three scenarios, the attributable risks show that the effect of the exposure is much greater in Scenario A than Scenario B, and even less so in Scenario C where the underlying risk is quite low. Although the risk of outcome is doubled in individuals exposed in all three scenarios, the absolute risk of outcome in those exposed increases by 10% in Scenario A, 5% in scenario B, but only 1% in Scenario C.

Feedback on Activity 3.5

For Scenario A, the attributable fraction is $(20 - 10) \div 20 = 0.50$. For Scenario B, the attributable fraction is $(10 - 5) \div 10 = 0.50$. And for Scenario C, the attributable fraction is $(2 - 1) \div 2 = 0.50$. For all three scenarios: 50% of the outcome among individuals exposed can be attributed to the exposure and 50% is the background risk, which may be due to other risk factors.

Feedback on Activity 3.6

1. The population attributable risk of exposure to chronic hepatitis B is $94 - 4 = 90$ per 100,000 person-years. This can be interpreted as follows: 90 liver cancer cases per 100,000 person-years in this population can be attributed to chronic hepatitis B infection.
2. The population attributable fraction is $(94 - 4) \div 94 = 0.96$, so 96% of liver cancer cases in the population are attributable to chronic hepatitis B infection, and could be avoided if hepatitis B infection were to be eliminated from the population

Feedback on Activity 3.7

1. An appropriate measure to assess the strength of an association in this example would be the incidence rate ratio (IRR) because we are given

the incidence rate in each group. The IRR of lung cancer mortality in smokers compared with non-smokers = 140 ÷ 10 = 14.00. The IRR of ischaemic heart disease (IHD) mortality in smokers compared with non-smokers = 669 ÷ 413 = 1.62. [*Note*: You could have said risk ratio, and this would have produced the same result because the denominators are standardized. However, the underlying measure is a rate, not a risk.]

2. An IRR of 14.00 for the association of smoking with lung cancer mortality compared with an IRR of 1.62 for the association of smoking with IHD mortality indicates that smoking is much more strongly associated with lung cancer mortality than it is with IHD mortality.

3. To calculate how many deaths per year can be attributed to cigarette smoking, we need to calculate the attributable risk for each disease by subtracting the incidence rate in unexposed individuals from that in exposed individuals. The attributable risk for lung cancer = 140 − 10 = 130 deaths per 100,000 person-years. The attributable risk for IHD = 669 − 413 = 256 deaths per 100,000 person-years. Although the IRRs show that the association between lung cancer mortality and cigarette smoking is stronger, a greater number of deaths from IHD can be attributed to cigarette smoking. [*Note*: We cannot calculate the population attributable risk because we do not have population-level data.]

4. To calculate the proportion of deaths due to cigarette smoking, we need to calculate the attributable fraction. The attributable fraction for lung cancer deaths is (140 − 10)/140 = 0.93 or 93%. The attributable fraction for IHD deaths is (669 − 413)/669 = 0.38 or 38%. This means that 93% of lung cancer deaths and 38% of IHD deaths among cigarette smokers are due to cigarette smoking, if we assume that cigarette smoking is causally related to lung cancer and IHD deaths.

Interpreting associations 4

Overview

Epidemiological measures of association between an exposure and outcome cannot be used to infer causality unless alternative explanations have been excluded. In this chapter, you will learn about alternative explanations for an apparent association between an exposure and an outcome: chance, bias, and confounding. The role of these effects needs to be considered when designing a study, and assessed whenever an association is found. Finally, to infer causality, it is necessary to build up supportive evidence, for example by using the Bradford Hill guidelines for causality.

Learning objectives

When you have completed this chapter, you should be able to:

- explain the concept of chance for measures of frequency and association
- describe how selection bias and information bias may distort associations
- identify potential confounders and how to control for their effects in analysis
- describe methods for avoiding chance, bias, and confounding in study design
- distinguish between statistical association and causality
- apply the guidelines for evaluating causality

Critical appraisal

The aim of analytical epidemiology is to determine whether there is an association between an exposure and outcome, and whether this is causal (i.e. the exposure is at least partially responsible for the outcome) and could provide a target for public health interventions. In Chapter 3, you learned about measures of association and the need to assume causality to estimate the impact of an exposure. However, before we can infer causality, it is necessary to critically appraise the evidence and exclude other possible reasons for a measured association. The three main alternative explanations for an observed epidemiological association are **chance**, **bias**, and **confounding**. Once these have been excluded, we must consider whether there is sufficient evidence that an association is likely to be causal.

Chance (random error)

It is usually not feasible to measure the outcome and/or exposure in every member of a given population or subgroup, so we make inferences about a population from a sample of individuals. Perhaps we want to know the number of children who have received three doses of diphtheria-tetanus-pertussis (DTP3) vaccine, as a marker of access to routine child health interventions. If we question the mothers of 10 infants at random, and then repeat this several times for different infants, we would most likely get a different number with full DTP3 coverage each time. This is known as sampling variation, caused by random error or 'chance'.

If we took 100 random samples of 10 infants from a population where the 'true' DTP3 coverage was 60%, we would most frequently measure values close to the true value, and less frequently measure values much lower or higher by chance. This is known as a sampling distribution, and most random variables tend to show a distribution this shape, also known as a bell-shaped curve or 'normal distribution' (see Figure 4.1).

This sampling distribution forms the basis for statistical inference, indicating how representative of the population a sample result is, i.e. the **probability** of obtaining a true result versus a false result. Figure 4.1 represents two sampling distributions we might see if we repeated the sample hundreds of times with different individuals. The height and width of the curve will change with the amount of variation in the value being

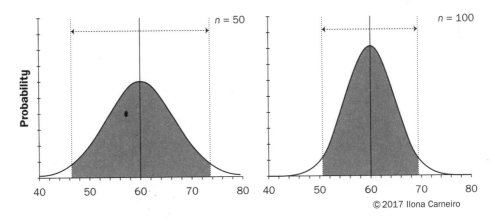

© 2017 Ilona Carneiro

Figure 4.1 Hypothetical sampling distribution curves for a sample of 50 versus 100 individuals

Note: The vertical solid line denotes the true population value; the shaded area under the curve, delimited by the dotted arrow, identifies the 95% confidence interval.

measured. Figure 4.1 shows the distribution for a sample of 50 infants on the left compared with 100 infants on the right. As the number of observations increases, the sample becomes more representative of the population of interest: the probability of measuring the true value increases and the variability decreases. Increasing **sample size** is the main way to reduce the role of chance observations in an epidemiological study.

In analytical epidemiology, we calculate relative risk as a measure of difference in the frequency of outcome between the exposed and unexposed groups. We want to know whether the observed relative risk from our study sample is representative of the underlying study population. This information is provided by two measures from statistical tests: the P-value and confidence interval.

The **P-value** is the probability that a measure (e.g. mean, proportion, frequency) from a sample occurred by chance, and that it does *not* exist in the population from which the sample was selected. The smaller the P-value, the stronger the evidence that the observed value is real. A P-value of 0.05 indicates a 5% probability the observation occurred by chance, and anything below this is generally considered low enough to imply that the result is not due to chance. However, this should not be used as a fixed threshold for reporting **statistical significance**, as there is little difference between a P-value of 0.04 and 0.06. Results in this range should be reported as *borderline* statistically significant, perhaps requiring further investigation. Whatever the P-value, we need to consider whether the magnitude of the effect would be of clinical or public health importance, and must look at the plausible range of values given by the confidence interval.

The **confidence interval** is a range of values, estimated from a sample, which includes the 'true' population value based on a predefined probability (usually 95%, but occasionally 90% or 99%). In Figure 4.1, if the total area under the curve represents the results of 100 repeated samples of DTP3 coverage, the shaded area represents the expected results from 95 of these samples. The values at either end of this shaded area are known as the limits of the confidence interval (CI). In Figure 4.1, the smaller sample size would give us 95% confidence that the true DTP3 coverage in the population is between 46.4% and 73.6%, while the larger sample of 100 individuals gives a narrower 95% CI of 50.4–69.6%. The larger sample is more representative of the true population, and the narrower CI indicates a more precise estimate. Values outside the CI (represented by the unshaded 'tails' of the curve in Figure 4.1) are not impossible to observe, but are less probable. There is a 5% probability of sampling values outside the 95% CI (2.5% in either tail), and this relates directly to the P-value.

For a relative risk (prevalence ratio, odds ratio, risk ratio, incidence rate ratio) where the value 1.00 represents no association, if the 95% CI does not include 1.00, we can say that the association is significant at the 5% level. This is because there is less than 5% chance that there is no association, so $P < 0.05$. Confidence intervals for relative risks are not symmetrical about the RR, as they are calculated on a logarithmic scale and then back-transformed.

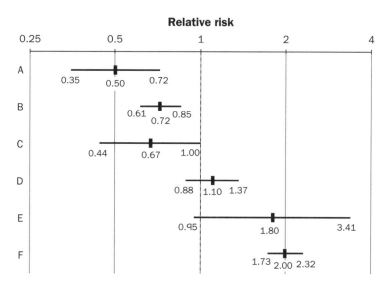

Figure 4.2 Relative risks (shown by the central vertical markers) and 95% confidence intervals (horizontal lines) from six studies (A–F)

Note: Confidence intervals appear symmetrical, as they are presented on a logarithmic scale.

If two 95% CIs do not overlap (e.g. Studies A and D in Figure 4.2), they are statistically significantly different from each other at $P < 0.05$. Note that the converse is not true, as there are some situations in which 95% CIs may overlap, yet the P-value could still be <0.05. Study A (Figure 4.2) shows a relative risk (RR) of 0.50 (95% CI: 0.35, 0.72), indicating that those in the exposed group had a 50% lower frequency of outcome than those in the unexposed group. As the upper limit of the 95% CI is far from 1.00, we can say that this association is highly significant at the 5% probability level.

🖋 **Activity 4.1**

Figure 4.2 shows the relative risks and 95% CIs from six analytical studies. For studies B–F, describe what the results show and indicate whether the finding is statistically significant.

Bias (systematic error)

While chance deals with random error due to sampling variability, bias is a systematic (i.e. non-random) error that leads to a deviation from the truth. Figure 4.3 represents the two types of error as hits on a target board, where the central circle represents the true measure. Board A shows a

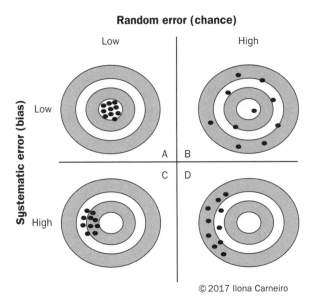

Figure 4.3 Representation of random versus systematic error

sample that reflects the true study population. Board B shows high random error, where by chance we may hit the target, or not. Board C shows a systematic error or bias towards an area to the left of the target. And Board D shows a bias to the left of the target, but with more random error than Board C, so that the data are less precise.

Sample size does not affect bias, and statistical methods cannot be used to adjust for bias, so it must be avoided through appropriate study design. Bias can be categorized as either selection bias or information bias.

Selection bias

Selection bias occurs when there is a systematic difference between the characteristics of individuals sampled and the population from which the sample is taken, or between comparison groups in a study. This can happen as a result of the definition of the study population and/or comparison groups, or because of missing or incomplete information. The **random selection** of study participants or **random allocation** of individuals to comparison groups aims to reduce systematic bias, but does not completely prevent it. To avoid any selection bias, it is important to clearly define the groups being compared.

In an **occupational cohort** study, for example, the overall health of the occupational cohort will usually be better than that of the general population, which includes individuals who are not well enough to work. This is known as the 'healthy worker effect', and can be reduced by selecting for comparison other workers without the exposure of interest. Even then, those who suffer most from an occupational exposure may be more likely to leave their jobs, resulting in the study selecting for those who are less affected.

Another example is membership of a group. People who choose to jog or attend a gym may be different in some other way to those who do not. Comparing regular exercisers with people who do not exercise regularly might indicate that exercise has excessive health benefits, although the two groups might also be different with respect to their diet or smoking habits.

Methods used to enumerate might also bias the selection of individuals. For example, in a study of access to routine health care using household lists drawn up by village elders, recent migrants or marginalized groups may be excluded from the study, making it less representative of the population as a whole.

Selection bias is an important issue in case-control studies, as cases and controls should differ only on the outcome of interest. As cases are often identified in a clinical setting, hospital-based controls are commonly used because it is logistically easier and avoids issues of differences between those who do and do not access health care. However, we need to be careful that the reason for admission to hospital is not potentially related to the exposure.

Inclusion and exclusion criteria can also affect the representativeness of a study if, for example, pre-screening of participants results in selecting those that are more likely to respond to a treatment or less likely to leave the study.

People who volunteer to participate in a study are 'self-selected' and are likely to differ from the general population in terms of health awareness, education, and other factors that may also affect the outcome of interest. Therefore, even if we are able to detect an association in a sample of volunteers, it does not mean it can be extrapolated to other populations, due to possible 'volunteer bias'.

Missing data can also affect the comparability of groups. For example, blood samples with insufficient volume for analysis are more likely to be those of individuals who are malnourished or dehydrated. Those who refuse to participate or respond to certain questions ('non-responders'), or who drop out of a study ('lost to follow-up'), may be different from those who contribute to the study as a whole, and this may vary between comparison groups. For example, individuals in an intervention study who receive an active intervention may be more likely to attend follow-up clinics if they feel a benefit compared with those receiving the placebo. If more cases are subsequently detected in intervention than in control individuals, we may wrongly conclude that the intervention has failed.

Information bias

Information bias (also known as **ascertainment bias**) occurs when the classification of exposure or outcome is inaccurate, and can be introduced by the investigators (observer bias), the study participants (responder bias) or measurement tools, such as weighing scales or questionnaires (**measurement bias**).

Observer bias (also **assessment bias**) refers to misclassification caused by the observer's knowledge of the comparison group. This may not be deliberate, or very large, but if it is systematically high or low, it can affect the study outcome. It may take the form of tending to 'round up' measures for one group and 'round down' measures for the other group. To reduce the effect of observer bias, the exposure status (or outcome status in a case-control study) should be concealed from the person measuring the outcome or exposure – this is known as **blinding**. It can also be reduced by all measurements either being undertaken by the same observers, or randomly by different observers.

Responder bias refers to systematic differences in the information provided by a study participant, and may take the form of recall, reporting or non-response bias. For example, in a case-control study of lung cancer and exposure to secondary smoke, cases may be more likely to remember their historical experience of secondary smoke (recall bias) if they are aware of the association between smoking and cancer, thereby overestimating the association. Similarly, in a study of sexual behaviour and prevalence of sexually transmitted infections (STIs), individuals with a higher number of sexual partners who are at higher risk of STIs may also be more likely to under-report their number of partners due to social stigma (reporting bias), resulting in an underestimate of the association. People who are less sexually active may choose not to answer questions they find embarrassing or intrusive (non-response bias).

We can reduce responder bias by 'blinding' study participants, which can be done using a **placebo** in intervention trials or concealing the hypothesis under investigation in other studies. For example, investigators may ask about a wide variety of exposures rather than focusing only on the exposure of interest. They may also ask a question in several different ways to ensure consistency of responses. To reduce recall bias, researchers can use objective records (e.g. vaccination cards) or shorten the recall period (e.g. asking 'Did you eat dairy products yesterday?' rather than 'Did you eat dairy products within the last week?'). Finally, by careful wording and piloting of questions beforehand, it is possible to reduce non-response bias.

Misclassification

Information bias may result in the misclassification of exposure or disease status in a non-differential (similar) or differential (distinct) way. Misclassification can affect the strength of association or lead to incorrect measures of association. Figure 4.4 shows how non-differential misclassification can lead to similar bias in both comparison groups, making them equally different from the true value, but not from each other. Differential misclassification results in bias in one group but not the other, giving the impression they are more different than they truly are.

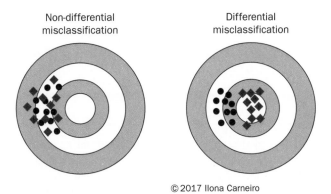

© 2017 Ilona Carneiro

Figure 4.4 Representation of non-differential and differential misclassification, where the central target represents the true value

Non-differential misclassification occurs when the two comparison groups (exposed/unexposed, cases/controls) are equally likely to be misclassified. Therefore, it is independent of exposure or outcome status, and will not alter the direction of any observed association. However, it may cause comparison groups to appear more similar than they are, leading to a bias towards no association or an *underestimation of the strength of the association*. We should consider the potential for non-differential misclassification when interpreting a study that shows no statistically significant association between the exposure and outcome.

Consider a case-control study of the association of oral contraceptive use with ovarian cancer, using 20 years' clinic records to determine exposure. It is unlikely that all records of oral contraceptive use over the previous 20 years from a family planning clinic will be traceable. The loss of records is likely to be distributed equally among cases and controls, since record-keeping in family planning clinics is independent of the risk of developing cancer. If the investigators decided to classify all women without a record as unexposed to contraceptives, then the odds of exposure would be underestimated in both cases and controls. This would lead to underestimation of the effect of contraceptives on ovarian cancer.

Differential misclassification occurs when classification of the exposure is dependent on the outcome or vice versa, and is generally due to observer or responder bias. It can lead to the overestimation or underestimation of a measure of association, and may also lead to false associations. For example, in a case-control study of lung cancer in smokers, if the exposure to tobacco smoke was determined by questioning the study participants, there may be a tendency for recall or reporting bias. Cases that are heavy smokers may underestimate their consumption because of the social stigma, leading to an underestimate of the association. Alternatively, given public knowledge of the association, cases may be more likely to blame their disease on tobacco exposure and report past consumption more accurately, while controls may have poorer recollection and underestimate past exposure, leading to an overestimate of the association.

✎ Activity 4.2

A survey of a prospective cohort of nurses asked them to categorize their natural hair colour and their skin tanning ability on a scale of none to dark. A case-control study of skin melanoma was conducted within the same cohort several years later and they were surveyed again. In the second survey, the responses for hair colour were the same, but some newly identified melanoma cases reported a reduced skin tanning ability compared with their original responses. The pre-existing cases and controls did not change their reported tanning ability between the two surveys.

1. Identify what type of bias may be present in this study of the association between skin tanning ability and melanoma.
2. Explain how this could affect the study findings.

Confounding

Confounding is a key concept in epidemiology that occurs when an apparent association between an exposure and an outcome is distorted by another independent factor (**confounder**). Once the confounding effect is adjusted for, there may be no association, or the measure of association may be different. For example, an association between occupation and lung cancer could be partly due to the occupational cohort being more likely to smoke, or smokers being more likely to choose a specific occupation, thus putting them at increased risk of lung cancer. A confounder may either have a direct causal association with the outcome or it may act as a proxy measure for unknown causes, such as age and socio-economic status. A confounding factor must be *independently* associated with both the exposure and the outcome, and must *not* be on the **causal pathway** between the two.

If a factor is on the causal pathway between the exposure and outcome – that is, the exposure leads to a factor that causes the outcome – it is not a confounder. For example, coronary heart disease is associated with high blood cholesterol, which is a direct result of diet. Blood cholesterol does not provide an *alternative explanation* for a relationship between diet and coronary heart disease, but is an intermediary between the two, and is therefore a 'mediator' rather than a confounder.

✎ Activity 4.3

A prospective cohort study in the USA of more than 400,000 people aged 50–70 years looked at the relationship between reported coffee drinking and all-cause mortality. It found that people who drank six or more cups of coffee per day had a relative risk of dying of 1.50 compared with those who did not drink coffee. However, after adjusting for several factors, the 'adjusted' relative risk of dying in this study population was 0.90.

1. What is your interpretation of the initial 'crude' relative risk result?
2. Provide your interpretation of the 'adjusted' relative risk result, and explain the difference.
3. List some factors for which the study authors may have adjusted.

Dealing with confounding

To observe the true effect of an exposure on an outcome, we need to avoid or control for confounding. There are three ways to avoid confounding when designing a study:

1. **Randomization** involves the random allocation of individuals to exposure and control groups, such that each study participant has an equal chance of being exposed or unexposed. If the sample size is sufficiently large, this method ensures the equal distribution between exposure groups of known and *unknown* confounders. This is the best method to avoid confounding, but can only be used in intervention studies.
2. **Restriction** limits the study to people who are similar in relation to the confounder. For example, if sex is known to be a confounder, the study might only include men. However, this means that the results of the study cannot then be extrapolated to women.
3. **Matching** selects two comparison groups to have the same distribution of potential confounders, and is generally only used in case-control studies. At an individual level, it is known as 'pair matching'. For example, when looking at the effect of hygiene practices on the risk of diarrhoea, a community control of the same age is identified for each diarrhoea case. At a group level, it is called 'frequency matching'. For example, when looking at exposure to smoking, female cases of lung cancer may be matched to female hospital controls and male cases matched to male controls.

There are two ways to control for confounding when analysing a study, if data on confounders have been measured:

1. **Stratification** is an extension of frequency matching, as it measures the association between exposure and outcome separately for each

category (stratum) of a confounder. For example, in a study of the association between long-term cannabis use and cognitive function, the measure of association should be calculated separately for each age group, as age is likely to be associated with amount of cannabis exposure and independently with cognitive function. The results can then be combined to obtain a measure of association that has been *adjusted* for the effects of the confounder. Always try to limit the number of strata in the analysis, as the sample size of each stratum will be reduced, increasing the role of chance.

2. **Statistical modelling** allows us to adjust simultaneously for several confounders using methods such as multivariate **regression** analyses (see Chapter 5).

Our ability to control for confounding will depend on the accuracy with which potential confounders have been measured. Non-differential (random) misclassification of a confounder would underestimate the effect of that confounder, reducing our ability to control for it. This is known as **residual confounding** and it *biases* the association between the exposure and outcome in the same direction as the confounding.

For example, a case-control study found that laryngeal cancer was associated with a four times greater odds of regular alcohol consumption (odds ratio = 4.22) (Becher, 1992). After adjusting for the confounding effect of smoking (i.e. comparing smokers to non-smokers), this was reduced slightly to give an odds ratio of 4.02. However, after adjusting for the average number of cigarettes smoked per day, which is a more precise measurement, the odds ratio reduced to 3.07. This shows that using only two categories of smoking resulted in residual confounding, because it was not a sufficiently accurate measure of exposure to smoking to be able to adjust for the confounding effect.

Effect modification

If a factor results in a varying association between exposure and outcome for different subgroups, this is known as **interaction** or **effect modification**. An effect modifier can be on the causal pathway. For example, cigarette smoking causes lung cancer, but the mortality rate is higher in women than in men, even when smoking intensity is accounted for. In this case, sex is an *effect modifier* in the relationship between cigarette smoking and lung cancer, and it would be misleading to calculate an overall estimate of effect for men and women combined. Effect modification is a natural occurrence that needs to be described, not controlled for, so separate measures of effect must be presented. With confounding, the stratified measures of association will differ from the crude measure, but they will be similar across strata. However, for effect modification, the measures of association will differ across strata, so separate measures must be calculated and presented.

Activity 4.4

Consider a hypothetical study aimed at measuring the association between helminth (intestinal worm) infection and cognitive ability. Five hundred children aged 7–16 years took age-appropriate tests of learning, memory, and other factors, and were subsequently tested for helminth infection. Of 250 infected children, 75 had adequate cognitive ability and 175 had a poor result. Of 250 uninfected children, 175 did adequately and 75 did poorly.

1. Draw up a 2 × 2 table from these results and calculate a prevalence ratio for the effect of helminth infections on cognitive ability in this study.
2. Tables 4.1 and 4.2 present the results by age group. Calculate the prevalence ratio for each age group and compare your results with those for question (1). How would you interpret this?

Table 4.1 Data on cognitive ability by helminth infection status for 7–11-year-olds

	Cognitive ability		
Helminth infection	Poor	Adequate	Total
Yes	150	50	200
No	25	75	100
Total	175	125	300

Table 4.2 Data on cognitive ability by helminth infection status for 12–16-year-olds

	Cognitive ability		
Helminth infection	Poor	Adequate	Total
Yes	25	25	50
No	50	100	150
Total	75	125	200

Inferring causality

Once we have discounted or adjusted for alternative explanations of an apparent epidemiological association, we must look to the meaning of this association. A statistically significant association between an exposure and an outcome does not imply causality. For example, in a *baseline* survey of 10,000 children, of whom half were subsequently randomized to receive an intervention, the mean haemoglobin concentration was significantly different (11.7 vs 11.9 g/dL). The groups are very large, have been randomized, and no interventions have yet been applied. There is therefore no explanation for any association between the randomization group and mean haemoglobin. In addition, the magnitude of difference is very small; it is only statistically significant because of the fine grading of the measurement, low variability between children, and the large sample size. We therefore should apply our judgement as to whether a statistically significant result has epidemiological or clinical importance, and whether there is a logical basis for an observed association.

Sir Austin Bradford Hill (Hill, 1965) listed nine considerations that are often used in epidemiology to gather evidence for a causal relationship:

1. *Temporality* – while it may seem obvious that the exposure *must* be present or have occurred prior to the outcome, this may be difficult to assess for slowly developing outcomes. For example, does diet lead to a digestive disorder, or do the unrecognized **symptoms** of the disorder affect the sufferer's diet? Temporality is also not easy to establish in cross-sectional or case-control studies, where the exposure and outcome are measured simultaneously. In such cases, an apparent risk factor could be a consequence of the outcome, which is known as **reverse causality**.
2. *Strength* – the stronger the association between the exposure and outcome, the less likely that the relationship is due to some other factor. For example, 10 times greater odds of laryngeal cancer among heavy alcohol drinkers decreases the likelihood that the relationship is wholly confounded by some other factor. A confounder would have to be much more frequent among heavy drinkers than non-drinkers. This criterion does not imply that an association of small magnitude cannot be causal, but it is more difficult to exclude alternative explanations in such cases.
3. *Consistency* – or repeatability. If the same association has been observed from various studies and in different geographic settings, it suggests that the association is real. For example, the assessment of a cause–effect relationship between cigarette smoking and coronary heart disease has been enhanced by similar results having been obtained by several cohort and case-control studies conducted over 30 years in different populations.
4. *Dose–response* – is there an increased risk of outcome with increased exposure? For example, the increased risk of lung cancer among heavy smokers compared with moderate smokers, and the increased risk among moderate smokers compared with light smokers. However, a dose–response relationship alone does not confirm causality and the absence of a dose–response relationship does not rule out causality.
5. *Plausibility* – the existence of a reasonable biological mechanism for the cause and effect lends weight to the association, but depends on existing knowledge. For example, a causal relationship between the moderate consumption of alcohol and decreased risk of coronary heart

disease is enhanced by the fact that alcohol is known to increase the level of high-density lipoprotein, which is associated with a decreased risk of coronary heart disease. However, the lack of a known or postulated mechanism does not necessarily rule out a cause–effect relationship. For example, John Snow hypothesized that water was the source of cholera epidemics in London long before the identification of *Vibrio cholera* (see Chapter 1).

6. *Reversibility* – relates to whether an intervention to remove or reduce the exposure results in the elimination or reduction of the outcome. For example, vitamin D deficiency is associated with muscle weakness, and older people are prone to develop vitamin D deficiency. However, it is difficult to infer a causal association between vitamin D deficiency and muscle weakness in the elderly. Other conditions may also cause weakness or tiredness, preventing elderly people from going outside and being exposed to sunlight (a source of vitamin D), and thus confound the association. Randomized intervention trials of vitamin D supplementation in the elderly have shown that it improves muscle strength and function, indicating causality (Janssen et al., 2002).

7. *Coherence* – refers to a logical consistency with other information. For example, the simultaneous increase in smoking habits and incidence of lung cancer over time supported a causal link, and the isolation from cigarette smoke of factors that caused cancer in laboratory animals further contributed to this (Hill, 1965).

8. *Analogy* – similarity with other established cause–effect relationships helps to support the argument for causality. For example, previous experience with the effects of thalidomide or rubella infection in pregnancy would lend support for a causal effect of another drug or viral infection in pregnancy with similar, but weaker, evidence.

9. *Specificity* – relates to the relationship being specific to the outcome of interest. For example, if a study of the effect of bicycle helmets showed a reduction only in head injuries and not those to other parts of the body, it would strengthen the inference of a protective effect of the helmet, and reduce the likelihood that the association was confounded by factors such as helmet-wearers being more careful riders (Weiss, 2002). However, many outcomes are the result of more than one exposure (see pp. 13–14). For example, smoking is a cause of coronary heart disease, but high cholesterol is also a cause of coronary heart disease, while smoking is also a cause of lung cancer and other illnesses.

✎ **Activity 4.5**

The cause of Alzheimer's – a neurodegenerative disease associated with old age – remains unknown. A recent study examined brain tissue from 27 cadavers and found evidence of fungal cells in all 16 people who had

Alzheimer's disease when they were alive, but none in the remaining 11 who had not had Alzheimer's disease (Pisa et al., 2015). Using the information given, what evidence is there for or against a causal relationship between fungal infection and Alzheimer's disease?

Conclusion

In this chapter, you have been introduced to alternative explanations for measured epidemiological associations: chance, bias, and confounding. These effects need to be considered when designing an epidemiological study, and evaluated when reviewing epidemiological data. We have also reviewed the type of evidence necessary to support a causal association, which is key to calculating measures of impact, and developing appropriate public health interventions.

This is the end of Section 1 and you should now have a foundation in the principles of epidemiology. In Section 2, you will focus more on the design and interpretation of descriptive and analytical research studies. This will allow you to consolidate what you have learned so far, and to expand your understanding of the research applications of epidemiology.

Additional activities to test your understanding

✎ Activity 4.6

A randomized, clinical intervention trial compared the effect of miltefosine, the first oral drug for the treatment of zoonotic cutaneous leishmaniasis caused by *Leishmania major*, with a standard treatment. The outcome of interest was clinical recovery (cure) measured 3 months post-treatment, when 21 of 25 patients who received oral miltefosine were cured and 16 of 25 patients who received the standard treatment were cured.

1. Calculate and interpret the risk ratio to compare treatment results after 3 months, using the control group as baseline. How would you interpret this?
2. The investigators calculated a 95% confidence interval (95% CI) of 0.93–1.84 and *P*-value of 0.11 for this risk ratio. Interpret what the 95% CI and *P*-value shown for this study tell you.
3. How might you reduce the role of chance in this study?

✎ Activity 4.7

A cross-sectional study was conducted to assess the association between a school-based health promotion package and adolescents' use of health services in District Y of northern Ghana. The investigators were interested in exposure to school-based health promotion activities. Participants were selected randomly from 'exposed' students attending the 10 schools in which the health promotion package had been implemented for the previous 2 years, and 'unexposed' students attending 10 schools that had not implemented the package. The outcome of interest was the prevalence of self-reported attendance at health services in the previous year measured through a survey undertaken at the schools.

1. Could measurement of exposure introduce bias into this study? Give reasons for your answer.
2. Could measurement of the study outcome introduce bias into this study? Give reasons for your answer.

✎ Activity 4.8

An intervention study of 1000 women of different ages showed a strong association between intense exercise and reduced risk of osteoporosis.

1. Define the concept of confounding in the context of this study.
2. Describe how this study finding could be the result of confounding.
3. How could you address potential confounding in this study?

Feedback on activities in Chapter 4

Feedback on Activity 4.1

1. For Study B, the relative risk (RR) = 0.72 (95% CI: 0.61, 0.85), indicating a 28% lower frequency of outcome in the exposed group, i.e. the exposure is protective. As the 95% CI does not overlap with 1.00, this association is significant at the 5% probability level.
2. For Study C, the RR = 0.67 (95% CI: 0.44, 1.00), indicating a 33% lower frequency of outcome in the exposed group. As the upper limit of the

95% CI is 1.00, there is a borderline statistically significant association. (In fact, the *P*-value will probably be 0.05.)

3. For Study D, the RR = 1.10 (95% CI: 0.88, 1.37). As the 95% CI includes 1.00, this indicates no statistically significant association between the exposure and outcome.

4. For Study E, the RR = 1.80 (95% CI: 0.95, 3.41), indicating 80% increased frequency of outcome in the exposed group compared with the unexposed group. However, as the CI includes 1.00, this is not statistically significant at the 5% probability level. (Given the magnitude of effect and the wide CI, this would warrant further investigation with a larger sample size.)

5. For Study F, the RR = 2.00 (95% CI: 1.73, 2.32), indicating twice as much frequency of outcome in the exposed group. As the 95% CI is far away from 1.00, we can say that this association is highly significant at the 5% probability level.

Feedback on Activity 4.2

1. There was reporting bias in the case-control study. Those diagnosed with melanoma since the previous survey subsequently reported their skin-tanning ability to be lower than that prior to diagnosis. This was a form of differential misclassification, as it occurred in only one outcome group (cases), and affected the classification of their exposure. [This was described by the study authors as a systematic shift in self-reported exposure after the outcome had occurred (Weinstock et al., 1991).]

   You may have said that this was an occupational cohort of nurses, so there could be some selection bias if nurses differ from the general population with regards to their incidence risk or rate of skin melanoma. This could affect the applicability of the study results to the general population. However, the association between melanoma and skin-tanning ability was measured using a case-control study design, and both cases and controls were nurses from the same cohort, so this would not lead to selection bias within the case-control study.

2. If the cases underestimated their skin-tanning ability after diagnosis, perhaps because they thought this was the cause of their melanoma, then this could bias the result towards a greater association between poor tanning ability and melanoma than truly existed. However, there was no objective measure of skin-tanning ability, so it is also possible that the cases had overestimated their skin-tanning ability in the first survey, and their melanoma diagnosis made them aware that their skin was truly more sensitive. If the reported exposure to reduced tanning in cases was more accurate in the second survey, then this could give an unbiased answer. It is not possible to determine with certainty how reporting bias may have affected the results.

Feedback on Activity 4.3

1. The crude relative risk of 1.5 suggests that people who drank six or more cups of coffee per day were 1.5 times or 50% more likely to die during the study period than those who did not drink as much coffee.
2. The adjusted relative risk suggests that people who drank six or more cups of coffee per day were 0.90 times or 10% less likely to die during the study period than those who did not drink as much coffee. The difference between the two results suggests that the initial association was confounded by other factors. [*Note*: There is no statistical test to prove confounding; it is inferred by comparison of crude and adjusted measures.]
3. Factors that could affect mortality rates and may also be associated with coffee-drinking habits could be confounders. Possible confounders may include the following:

   - age – because all-cause mortality rates are known to vary by age, and between 50 and 70 years the mortality rate will be increasing with each additional year of age;
   - sex – because cause-specific mortality rates are known to vary between men and women;
   - ethnicity – because this may affect cause-specific mortality in the USA;
   - smoking status – because this is known to be a risk factor for many causes of death among older people in the USA;
   - alcohol consumption – because this is known to be a risk factor for many causes of death among older people in the USA.

Some other factors that the authors looked at in the real study included education, physical activity level, and consumption of red meat, fruits, and vegetables (Freedman et al., 2012).

Feedback on Activity 4.4

1. Your 2 × 2 table should look like Table 4.3.

Table 4.3 A 2 × 2 table of helminth infection status by cognitive ability score

Helminth infection	Cognitive ability		Total
	Poor	Adequate	
Yes	175	75	250
No	75	175	250
Total	250	250	500

In this study, the exposure is helminth infection and the outcome is cognitive ability. The prevalence of poor cognitive ability was 175 ÷ 250 = 70% among those infected with helminths and 75 ÷ 250 = 30% among those who were not infected. The prevalence ratio was (175÷250)/(75÷250) = 2.33, indicating that children infected with helminths were more than two times more likely to have poor cognitive ability than those uninfected.

2. Among 7–11-year-olds, the prevalence ratio was (150/200)/(25/100) = 3.00, indicating that children aged 7–11 infected with helminths in this study were three times more likely to have poor cognitive ability than uninfected children.

   Among 12–16-year-olds, the prevalence ratio was PR = (25/50)/(50/150) = 1.5, indicating that children aged 12–16 infected with helminths in this study were 1.5 times more likely to have poor cognitive ability than uninfected children.

   The initial (crude) prevalence ratio in part 1 is different from the prevalence ratios for the two age groups separately. If both age groups had similar results to each other, but were different from the combined results, we might conclude that age was a confounder. However, as the results are quite different for the two age groups, it suggests that age modifies the effect of helminth infection on cognitive ability, so age is an effect modifier.

Feedback on Activity 4.5

We can use the Bradford Hill criteria to examine the likelihood of causality, although there is not enough information given here to consider them all. The sample size is quite small but the strength of association between fungal infection of brain tissue and Alzheimer's is very strong, with 100% of cases being exposed and none of the controls being exposed. (As this is a case-control study design, we could calculate an odds ratio of exposure as (16 ÷ 0)/(0 ÷ 11) which cannot be mathematically defined.)

As this is a post-mortem study, we cannot say anything about temporality. We cannot tell whether the fungal infection gave rise to Alzheimer's, or whether the Alzheimer's enabled the fungal infection. This could be an example of reverse causality (Alzheimer's is thought to damage the blood–brain barrier).

Further studies would be needed to assess whether there is a causal link, the most definitive of which would be an intervention trial of antifungal drugs.

Feedback on Activity 4.6

1. The outcome is 'risk of recovery', i.e. the number of people that recovered during a fixed period of time. [*Note*: Although this is clinically known as a 'cure rate', in epidemiological terms it is a risk, as there is

no variation in person-time at risk.] The risk of recovery among the intervention group was 21 ÷ 25 = 0.84 or 84%. The risk of recovery among the control group was 16 ÷ 25 = 0.64 or 64%. Therefore, the risk ratio = (21 ÷ 25)/(16 ÷ 25) = 1.31.

A risk ratio of 1.31 indicates that those receiving miltefosine have a 31% higher likelihood of having achieved a cure at 3 months than those receiving standard treatment in this study. However, this does not tell us whether this difference is real or due to chance.

2. Evaluating the role of chance in study findings requires two related statistical assessments: (a) calculating a P-value to test the study hypothesis and determine the likelihood that sampling variability could explain the results; and (b) estimating the 95% CI to indicate the range within which the true result is likely to be.

A P-value of 0.11 is relatively high, indicating an 11% probability that the study result of 1.31 is due to chance. A 95% CI of 0.93–1.84 indicates that we can be 95% confident that the true risk ratio in the population from which the patients were drawn is between 0.93 and 1.84. Because this CI includes '1.00', we know that the P-value is greater than 0.05 and that the relative risk (RR) of 1.31 is not significant at the 5% level. The CI is relatively wide, so we could not be confident of extrapolating the observed RR estimate of 1.31 to the whole population.

3. Statistical significance and confidence intervals help to evaluate the role of chance as an alternative explanation of an observed association. The most common way of reducing the role of chance is to increase sample size, which decreases the P-value. The study sampled 50 participants, so a larger sample size might provide a more robust estimate.

Feedback on Activity 4.7

1. Yes, measurement of exposure to the health promotion package could cause bias in this study. We do not know what the promotion activities consisted of or whether there could be overlap ('**contamination**') between schools attended by participants categorized as 'exposed' and schools attended by participants categorized as 'unexposed'. For example, we do not know how far apart the health promotion and non-promotion schools were from each other. We also do not know if there were other activities to promote health service attendance in the communities from which the 'non-exposed' students were selected. The effect of such a bias would most likely *reduce the association* between outcome and exposure.

2. Yes, outcomes were measured through self-reporting, so information bias may have been introduced in the form of reporting bias. If 'exposed' students had been sensitized to the importance of attending health services, they might be more likely to report having attended in the past year. Additionally, one year is a long recall period and both 'exposed' and 'non-exposed' participants might not remember correctly whether they had attended services.

Feedback on Activity 4.8

1. The presence of confounding would mean that the observed association between exposure (intense exercise) and outcome (reduced osteoporosis risk) is due totally or in part to the effects of another variable or variables. Such a variable must be associated with intense exercise and independently associated with osteoporosis.

2. In this study, age could act as a confounder, providing an alternative explanation for the observed association between heavy exercise and osteoporosis risk. Young women, as a group, tend to exercise more intensely. Additionally, and independently, younger women have a lower risk of osteoporosis. [*Note*: This alternative association does not need to be causal – increased age does not necessarily cause osteoporosis.]

3. The three common ways of controlling for confounding at the design stage are randomization, restriction, and matching. As this is an intervention study, the intervention and control groups could have been frequency-matched by age group, prior to randomization to reduce residual confounding by age within these groups. Confounding can also be addressed at the analysis stage: the results could be stratified by age group, or adjusted for individual age in a multivariate regression analysis, if the sample size is sufficiently large.

SECTION 2

Epidemiological research studies

Study design and analysis 5

Overview

An epidemiological investigation starts by identifying the association of interest and choosing an appropriate study design. Investigators use methods to reduce the role of chance, bias, and confounding, and collect data (information) in a way that will maximize its utility. In this chapter, you will learn the importance of choosing an appropriate study design, developing a protocol, and managing data. Design-specific topics will be covered in subsequent chapters. You will also be introduced to data analysis, and the interpretation of common statistics presented in epidemiological reports.

Learning objectives

When you have completed this chapter, you should be able to:

- identify the principal epidemiological study designs
- outline the steps for developing a study protocol
- evaluate the role of different sampling strategies in obtaining representative data
- recognize different data types and how best to report them
- describe the basic approaches to analysing and interpreting epidemiological data

Study designs

Chapter 1 introduced descriptive and analytical sources of epidemiological data, both of which are observational. Descriptive data provide information on the *frequency* and distribution of an *outcome* or *exposure*, but do not analyse the association between them. Analytical studies measure the *association* between an exposure and outcome, with the aim of inferring causality. Intervention studies also measure the association between exposure and outcome, but the investigators allocate the exposure. Figure 5.1 shows a flowchart that identifies the key properties of different epidemiological study designs, and can be used to distinguish between them.

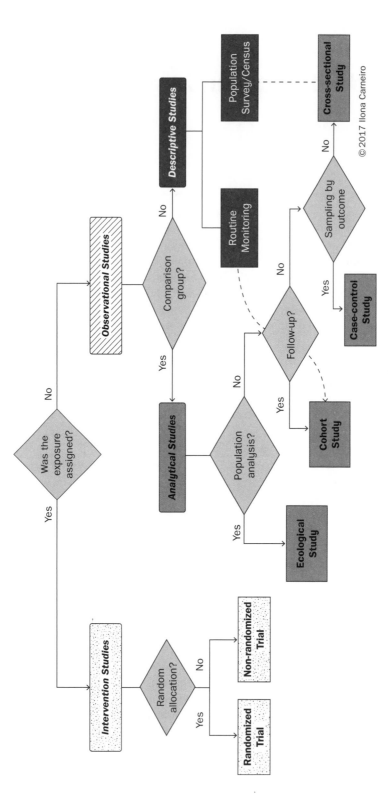

Figure 5.1 Flowchart to identify an epidemiological study design

Note: Diamonds indicate points of differentiation, rectangles with rounded corners denote categories of design, and rectangles with square corners denote different study types. Dashed lines show overlap between descriptive and analytical methods.

Source: Based on Grimes and Schulz (2002).

©2017 Ilona Carneiro

Descriptive studies

Descriptive studies are used to identify whether the burden of an outcome is of public health importance, or as part of a situation analysis for further investigation. For example, the 15-fold increase in routinely recorded lung cancer deaths in England and Wales between 1922 and 1947 prompted a call for studies to investigate the cause of this (Doll and Hill, 1950). Descriptive studies may use data from:

- censuses and population surveys;
- routine monitoring systems such as vital registration of births and deaths, registries of notifiable outcomes and health facility data;
- cross-sectional 'prevalence' surveys; or
- outbreak investigations.

Analytical studies

There are four main types of observational analytical study:

1. Ecological studies compare the frequency (prevalence or incidence) of outcome and exposure at a *population level*. They may identify epidemi-ological associations that then require further investigation to infer causality. Using the lung cancer example above, mortality rates differed between urban and rural populations, lending support to the hypothesis that the risk factor may be atmospheric pollution.
2. Cross-sectional studies compare the *prevalence* of outcome with expos-ure status at one time point from a random sample of individuals. These are rapid and less costly than other studies and may be best for com-mon or chronic outcomes. The simultaneous collection of outcome and exposure data makes it difficult to infer causality; these studies are often used to provide preliminary evidence of an individual-level associ-ation, e.g. population surveys of obesity and reported dietary habits.
3. Cohort studies compare the *incidence* of outcome in individuals with recorded differences in exposure. These require a well-defined popula-tion and are usually time-consuming, costly, and logistically more difficult than other study designs. However, they are ideal for inferring causality, as the exposure is recorded prior to the outcome. For example, a large cohort of men working at several oil refineries could be followed up over several years to assess whether this occupation was associated with the incidence of various causes of death.
4. Case-control studies select individuals based on their outcome status and analyse whether they differ in relation to previous exposure, making these studies prone to selection and information bias. These are best for studying rare outcomes, or for outbreak investigations, where it would not be practical to follow up individuals over a long period. Early

case-control studies of AIDS (acquired immunodeficiency syndrome) identified risk groups and risk factors, resulting in the restriction of high-risk blood donors and promotion of safer behaviours even before identification of the human immunodeficiency virus (HIV) (Schulz and Grimes, 2002).

Intervention studies

Intervention studies allocate a protective exposure or remove exposure to a risk factor, and compare outcomes between exposed and unexposed individuals. This is the gold standard for inferring causality. Intervention studies may combine several study methods. For example, study of a malaria control intervention may start with a baseline descriptive cross-sectional study, followed by an analytical cohort study to analyse the effect on malaria incidence, and end with an analytical cross-sectional study to analyse the effect on malaria and anaemia prevalence.

✎ Activity 5.1

For each of the following examples, identify the study design used and list the possible measures of association that could be calculated:

1. A comparison of mobile phone usage in 50 people with brain cancer and 100 people without brain cancer.
2. A study of 10,000 people followed up over a 10-year period to identify the risk factors for heart disease.
3. A comparison of the prevalence of anaemia (haemoglobin < 8 g/dL) at 8 months' gestation among pregnant women given an insecticide-treated mosquito net to sleep under, compared with women given an untreated mosquito net to sleep under.
4. A comparison of national infant mortality rates by gross domestic product.
5. A survey of the number of children with existing *Ascaris lumbricoides* (an intestinal worm) infection and their household's access to running water.

Study protocol

When planning an epidemiological study, a study protocol is prepared to outline the methods to be used. The key components of any study protocol include: choice of study design, choice of study area and population, eligibility criteria for participants, sample size calculation, sampling methods, data collection approach and tools, statistical analysis of data, and ethics. It is important to detail these aspects of study design, ethical permission received, and conflicts of interest when reporting a study.

Guidelines and checklists have been published to encourage standardized reporting of epidemiological studies: Strengthening the Reporting of OBservational studies in Epidemiology (STROBE) for observational studies (www.strobe-statement.org), and Consolidated Standards of Reporting Trials (CONSORT) for intervention studies (www.consort-statement.org). The next sections cover the key aspects of a study protocol that need to be considered when planning or reviewing an epidemiological study.

Sampling

Epidemiological investigations are undertaken using a **sample population** (e.g. 500 infants attending vaccination clinics, 200 women over 55 years, 10 villages in Laos) and findings are then extrapolated to the **target population** (e.g. all infants in the country, women over 55 years in the UK, the population of Laos). In Chapter 4, you learned about the roles of chance and selection bias, and the need for the study sample population to be *representative* of the target population. We can reduce the role of chance by having a sufficiently large **sample size**. We can reduce selection bias by selecting a random sample from the study population, taking care to ensure that hard-to-reach or minority groups are proportionately sampled.

Sampling unit

First, we need to identify the unit of observation: individual, household, school, community, hospital, district, etc. The unit will often be determined by the level at which the exposure acts, although it is sometimes logistically easier to study groups. However, a comparison of improved cognitive function in 500 students taking omega-3 supplementation and 500 students taking a placebo is not the same as comparing it in five exposed schools and five unexposed schools each with 100 students. There are likely to be unmeasured similarities between students in the same school, and the sample size would need to be larger to account for this. This issue of group randomization is dealt with further in Chapter 8.

Eligibility criteria

The sample population should represent the general population for whom the results will be relevant. However, in some cases it is necessary to exclude certain individuals (e.g. those who could be harmed by participating, those who may be at greater risk of loss to follow-up). It is therefore important to develop clear **inclusion criteria** to specify the sample population of interest. For example, a study of diabetes in pregnancy may specify 'women enrolled in their first trimester of pregnancy' to obtain sufficient baseline data. **Exclusion criteria** specify those individuals who are not eligible for inclusion in the study, perhaps because they have underlying conditions that may interfere with assessment of the outcome. For example, in a study of the incidence of clinical malaria fevers, children with severe anaemia (haemoglobin < 5 g/dL) at baseline may be excluded because they require medical treatment and may be more prone to a severe outcome.

Sample size

Once we have identified our sampling unit and eligibility, it is necessary to define a specific, testable hypothesis. It is not sufficient to state the association of interest – for example: 'to measure the effect of gender on depression'. Instead, we must specify the comparison groups, expected size of the effect, and measure of frequency or association to be detected. This is known as the study objective and should explicitly mention subjects, study population, and magnitude of effect. For example: 'To detect a *30% difference* in the *prevalence* of *unipolar depression* between *men* and *women* in *British cities*.'

Two important concepts in sample size calculation are statistical **power** and **precision**. Statistical power is the probability of detecting an effect if it is real. Statistical precision is the probability of detecting an effect if it is *not* real, i.e. by chance (see *P*-values, p. 56). It is typical to aim for a sample size with 80–90% power and 5% precision (significance) to detect a valid estimate of effect. Increased statistical power and precision require increasingly larger sample sizes, and this will have implications for how much a study costs and how long it takes.

The size of effect to be detected will also determine the sample size. The larger the effect, the easier it is to detect and the fewer study subjects are required to obtain statistical significance. However, it is rare to find very large effects, so we need to decide what magnitude of effect would be of public health importance by undertaking a cost–benefit analysis. As the sample size increases, smaller differences will be detected as statistically significant, and we need to consider whether these differences are clinically important. If we found that people drinking one glass of orange juice per day reduced their risk of catching a cold by 50%, we might promote it or at least undertake more research into the nature of the relationship. However, if we found that one glass of orange juice a day reduced risk of a cold by only 10%, we would not necessarily recommend orange juice for everyone.

Sample size formulae vary with the outcome of interest (prevalence, incidence, mean) and the level of observation/intervention (individual, group). Formulae are available in several statistics textbooks (e.g. Kirkwood and Sterne, 2003), although computer statistical software packages (e.g. Stata, SPSS) are normally used for sample size calculation.

Sampling methods

To reduce selection bias, we should sample (i.e. select study participants from) the population with an equal probability of sampling any **subject** (e.g. individual, household, clinic). Random sampling usually requires a sampling frame (i.e. a list detailing all eligible subjects in the study population) from which to sample. If a sampling frame is difficult to obtain (e.g. in refugee camps or slums), a starting point may be selected at random, and then a bottle is spun and the fifth or tenth dwelling in that direction is also sampled, and the procedure is repeated until sufficient dwellings are recruited.

When a sampling frame is available, published tables of random numbers or computational random number generators are used to reduce selection bias. The following are some sampling approaches that may be used, although these may vary with the complexity of the study (e.g. if the population is spread out over a large area or if there are subgroups):

- *Simple random sampling* is **random selection** from the sampling frame; for example, labelling a different card for each district, shuffling them, and choosing the required number for the study.
- *Systematic sampling* is the selection of sampling units at regular intervals, rather than at random. This may be used when a fixed proportion (e.g. 20% of village households) is to be sampled.
- *Stratified sampling* is used when there are distinct groups or strata with different expected frequencies of the outcome or exposure of interest (e.g. age, gender, other potential confounders). To ensure that the sample represents the population, an equal proportion is sampled from each stratum using simple random sampling.
- *Cluster sampling* uses the hierarchical structure of the study population (e.g. region, district, village, hamlet) and samples all or most of those within the 'cluster'. For example, in an intervention study of the protective effect of insecticide-treated mosquito nets, where the intervention is known to protect other household members, x number of households (i.e. 'higher sampling unit' or 'cluster') would be sampled, and all eligible household members (i.e. 'primary sampling unit') within selected clusters would be included in the sample.
- *Multi-stage sampling* uses the hierarchical structure, but involves more than one stage of sampling. For example, in a study of school children (i.e. 'primary sampling unit'), x number of schools (i.e. 'higher sampling unit') will be randomly sampled from a regional list, and then y number of children will be randomly sampled from within each selected school. If the schools are of different sizes, then sampling is carried out using 'probability proportional to size', such that a school with three times as many pupils will be sampled three times more than another school.

Ethics and informed consent

The focus on ethical aspects of epidemiological research, such as minimizing risk to participants, obtaining informed consent, and protecting confidentiality, has increased significantly (Coughlin, 2006). Study proposals need to be submitted for ethical review by institutional and national bodies and ethical approval is necessary prior to commencing a research study – and sometimes before obtaining funding.

Before undertaking an epidemiological study, a case must be made for why the study itself, and its potential findings, may be beneficial to participants. Any potential benefits should also be distributed equally among the study participants, and across social groups. This is especially important for vulnerable populations, such as children, the elderly, and socio-economically disadvantaged subgroups. For example, a clinical trial of a novel HIV vaccine among children in a low-income country could not be justified if such a trial would not be granted ethical permission to be conducted in a high- or middle-income country.

For large-scale field studies, it is appropriate to inform local government and civil society. Community sensitization meetings may improve local understanding of the study aims and thus cooperation with investigators and recruitment to the study. Before participants are recruited into an epidemiological study, they must be made fully aware of what the study is about and what the potential risks and benefits are. Participants then freely choose to give their **consent** to participate. This is known as **informed consent**. It is important that individuals can refuse to participate and that consenting participants can drop out of the study at any time, without any adverse consequences for their access to preventive or treatment services.

Sometimes it is not possible for a participant to provide their consent – for example, in the case of a child or an unconscious patient – and in such cases consent must be obtained from a parent, caregiver or close relative. The information must be provided in the language of the consent giver and, if they are unable to read, all information must be clearly read to them. Consent usually takes the form of a signature, or a fingerprint for consent givers who cannot read. Details of the format of information and consent should be clearly stated when study results are reported.

✎ **Activity 5.2**

1. In a region of country X, all single births occurring in four randomly selected districts during a one-week period were identified from a birth register to assess the gender ratio. What do you think was the outcome measure, the type of sampling used, and the inclusion criteria?

2. In a large secondary school with nine classes of children aged 9–12 years, 100 girls were randomly selected from the class registers to be tested for rubella antibodies. What do you think was the outcome measure, the type of sampling used, and the inclusion criteria?
3. In country Y, six of 15 regions were randomly selected. Subsequently, 5% of households were selected from each of these six regions and a survey administered on access to health care among children under 5 years of age. What do you think was the outcome measure, the type of sampling used, and the inclusion criteria?

Data collection

The key to conducting a good epidemiological investigation is to plan the data collection and the analytical approach beforehand. Even studies with large sample sizes and unbiased subject selection can be seriously flawed if key data (e.g. confounders) are not collected. The methods used to collect the data will depend on the exposures and outcomes being studied and how practical and costly it is to collect them.

Routinely collected data on outcomes or exposures can often be obtained from medical records, census data, health surveys, cancer registries, and records kept by schools or employers. These *indirect data collection methods* have the advantage that the data are already available and can provide information relatively quickly and cheaply. However, quality may be poor due to missing or inaccurate data. Routine data systems are designed to serve objectives other than research, such as **surveillance**, and may not be able to provide all the information required. Therefore, a combination of data collection methods may be better.

Most epidemiological studies obtain data directly from the study participants (or their caregivers). *Direct data collection methods* include questionnaires (e.g. self-administered, filled in by an investigator), structured interviews (e.g. conducted face-to-face, by telephone), and clinical examination (e.g. having a blood sample taken for a diagnostic test). Data collection tools include questionnaires, specimen labels for clinical samples, and forms for clinical results. The advantage of direct data collection is that it is performed prospectively (even though questions may relate to historical events) and collection tools are designed for the specific study. However, in addition to being costly and time-consuming, there may be problems such as recall bias or a poor response rate.

Other types of data

Environmental data can also be collected, and advancements in global positioning system (GPS) technology enable us to identify the precise geographic location of a household, village or health centre. Specific data may be collected during an epidemiological study, or from routine sources of climate data (e.g. rainfall, cloud cover), or satellite images (e.g. land use, road access). Different layers of data (e.g. geographical, epidemiological) can be linked using geographic information systems (GIS) that connect the location of the data in space and time. This allows a more complex analysis of the data, enabling us to measure the incidence of childhood cancer in relation to distance to the nearest electricity pylon, or the prevalence of malaria infection in relation to altitude and rainfall, for example.

Social science research methods aim to explain the why or how of human behaviour, using different approaches to data collection. Structured interviews provide a framework for the interviewer, defining the wording and question sequence to improve the validity of responses. Other methods, such as semi-structured interviews, participant observation or focus group discussions, usually deal with limited numbers or non-randomly selected participants, making them inappropriate for the measurement of epidemiological associations. However, they are often useful as additional studies, and may explain why an association is or is not seen, depending on the complexity and sensitivity of the topic (for more on this subject, see Durand and Chantler, 2014).

Unique identifiers

Investigators must be able to link all necessary data to the appropriate study participant, using a relational database, which is a method of relating different layers of data. A study using multi-stage or cluster sampling will need to collect and link data on the different sampling levels. A cohort study will measure individuals repeatedly, including at least the baseline measurement and final contact recording the outcome. Names should not be used because, in addition to being common or misspelled, the identity of participants must be kept confidential and results reported anonymously.

Unique identifiers should be created for each sampling unit (e.g. individual, household, hospital) and used whenever data are collected. For example, a cohort study of malaria in children will define a unique identifier per child (e.g. number 00142) and then collect data on the child (e.g. name, date of birth, gender), the child's household (e.g. household size, distance to nearest health facility), and health facility visits (e.g. data on outpatient attendance, body temperature, haemoglobin level, presence of malaria parasites). Different data collection tools may be used for each layer of data, but all (e.g. household questionnaire, clinic record, blood slide) must record the same unique identifier that will enable, for example, a laboratory test result to be linked to the correct study participant.

Data management

It is important that data collection is standardized and investigators ensure the *validity* of the methods used (i.e. that they are measuring what they aim to measure). Data may be quantitative (numeric), qualitative (categorical) or open-ended, such as the comments from a focus group discussion in social science research. Data collection tools need to be carefully designed and piloted (pre-tested) to reduce errors.

Data format and legitimate values or ranges need to be defined when developing data collection tools and training people to collect the data. Data may be recorded on paper and entered on a computer, or may be directly input on a hand-held digital device. When data are being transferred from paper to a computer, it is advisable to double-enter the data to reduce data-entry inputting errors. The computer program should also be designed to restrict entry only to feasible response values, for example, prevent the entry of an age as '310' instead of '31' or a test result as anything other than 'positive', 'negative' or 'unknown'. The data should be regularly 'cleaned' to ensure that there are no impossible values (e.g. 50-year-old infants), to check for missing values, and to ensure that data can be linked (e.g. every participant enrolled has an outcome measure).

Data variables

The term 'variable' refers to data that can have more than one value, and is usually applied to each distinct unit of data that is collected. Quantitative variables are numerical and can be either discrete or continuous. Discrete variables have only a finite number of values and these cannot be subdivided meaningfully (e.g. number of mosquito nets owned). Continuous variables can take any value within a given range (e.g. blood pressure, age). Qualitative variables are categorical and include binary (e.g. Yes/No), ordered categorical (e.g. age groups), and unordered categorical data (e.g. religion).

Continuous variables can be grouped into categories, and categorical variables can be further grouped into binary variables. This increases the sample size in each category, providing greater *statistical power* to detect any effect. For example, haemoglobin concentration is a continuous variable, which might be grouped categorically as mild (10.0–10.9 g/dL), moderate (7.0–9.9 g/dL) or severe (<7.0 g/dL) anaemia. It can also be grouped binomially as moderately anaemic (<10 g/dL): Yes/No, for example. If social science methods are used to define outcomes or exposures (e.g. a case-control study of post-natal depression and a reported history of depression), these will need to be coded as binomial or categorical variables to measure the epidemiological association.

Activity 5.3

For each of the following analytical studies, identify: (i) the study design, (ii) outcome and exposure of interest, and (iii) whether the variables are binary, ordered or unordered categorical, or continuous. Indicate the appropriate measure of association and list potential confounders.

1. Investigators invited the caregivers of 500 children to participate in an epidemiological study by taking their children for testing for malaria parasites to a central point during a 5-day period. Caregivers were asked about the number of mosquito nets in the household, and for other information about the household.
2. Investigators surveyed 17,530 men working in the British civil service about their grade of employment (e.g. administrative, executive, clerical) and who were then followed up for 7½ years, during which there were 1086 deaths.
3. Investigators observed and – using a structured checklist – recorded whether the prescribing practice of 30 doctors to each of 10 patients with respiratory tract infections was consistent with national guidelines on antibiotic prescription. After 15 days, they conducted telephone interviews to ask patients whether their symptoms had resolved.
4. Using a structured questionnaire, investigators interviewed 80 women with breast cancer and their twin sisters without breast cancer about their previous history and length of oral contraception use.

Data reporting

Data presentation

Data are summarized by variable type. Binary and categorical variables may be summarized as proportions of the total (e.g. 49% male and 51% female). Continuous variables are usually presented as the average value of the variable and the amount of variation around this average.

Figure 5.2 shows three different types of data frequency distribution patterns. Most variables show a normal distribution (e.g. height); however, others are positively skewed, with the most values to the left and a 'tail' to the right (e.g. age with fewer people surviving to older ages), or negatively skewed, with most values to the right and a 'tail' to the left (e.g. period of gestation with most women carrying to full term and few premature births).

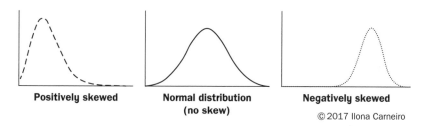

Figure 5.2 Data distribution patterns

These properties are used to identify the appropriate summary descriptors. A normally distributed variable can be summarized by its mean (sum of values divided by the number of values) and standard deviation, while a skewed variable can be summarized by its median (mid-point of ordered values) and interquartile range (25–75%, or middle 50% of ordered values). Such summary values are used to describe the baseline characteristics of a study sample, to compare exposed with unexposed groups, and to compare cases with controls.

Descriptive data may be presented graphically (Figure 5.3). In epidemiology, histograms are most commonly used to describe the distribution of a continuous variable, while bar charts are used to compare the means or proportional distribution for categorical variables.

Analytical data may also be presented graphically, most commonly as a scatterplot when investigating the relationship between two continuous variables (see Figure 5.4). If the relationship appears to be linear, we can draw a 'line of best fit' or 'trend line'. This is a straight line that best represents the data plotted and indicates the 'correlation' (relationship) between the two variables.

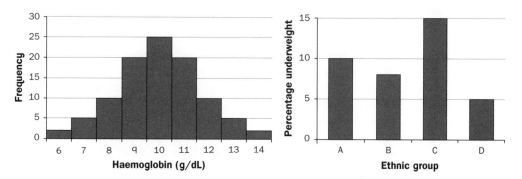

Figure 5.3 (a) Histogram of the frequency distribution of haemoglobin concentrations (g/dL) and (b) bar chart of the percentage of children underweight by ethnic group

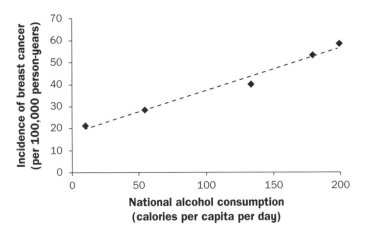

Figure 5.4 Scatterplot of national incidence of breast cancer per 100,000 person-years, by estimated per capita alcohol consumption for selected countries

Note: Diamonds denote countries and the dashed line shows the trend for selected data points.

Source: Adapted from Schatzkin et al. (1989).

✎ Activity 5.4

Using the information in Figure 5.4:

1. Identify the epidemiological study design, giving reasons for your answer.
2. Identify the exposure and outcome, specifying what type of data variables these are.
3. Describe the relationship shown between the outcome and exposure.

Data analysis

In addition to describing data, comparisons are made and relationships are tested using statistical techniques. These statistical methods are too complex to be covered in this book, but we will review some of the measures or terminology you may encounter in epidemiological reports. Statistical tests start with a **null hypothesis** that there is *no difference* between two measures (e.g. mean age between two groups, frequency between exposure and outcome groups). Descriptive data are compared using various statistical tests (e.g. *t*-tests for mean values, chi-squared tests for proportions). The result of these tests is the *P*-value, which represents the probability that a difference at least as big as the one observed could have occurred by chance alone, if there truly is no difference. A smaller *P*-value indicates a more significant ('true') result, but a larger value may be due to a lack of statistical power, and does not necessarily indicate that there is no difference (see Chapter 4). A low *P*-value may indicate a statistically significant difference, but this does not mean that

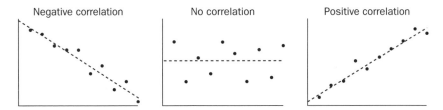

Figure 5.5 Scatterplots with trend lines showing different relationships of negative correlation (r < 0), no correlation (r = 0), and positive correlation (r > 0)

the difference is of clinical or research significance – for that we need to consider the magnitude of the difference.

Figure 5.4 shows how the relationship between two quantitative variables is compared using a trend line. The strength and direction of this relationship is described by the **correlation coefficient**. This is usually denoted as 'r' and can take any value between –1 and +1. If r is negative, it means that one variable decreases as the other increases (see Figure 5.5), while if it is positive, both variables increase together. The closer to +1 or –1 the coefficient is, the better the line fits the data (the closer the data points are to the line), indicating a stronger association. The closer to zero, the weaker the association, so that $r = 0$ means that the variables are not associated.

Regression models

In Chapter 3, we calculated measures of association for the effect of interest, when we had two categories of exposure. For more categories, we calculated the association separately between each category and the reference. If we want to compare multiple categories or look at a continuous exposure, we can use a more complex statistical method known as regression analysis, using computer software. While correlation measures the strength and direction of association, regression uses a mathematical model to describe how the variables are related and to predict the outcome (for further information, see Kirkwood and Sterne 2003).

Continuous variables, such as blood pressure or haemoglobin concentration, may be analysed using linear regression, with the results presented as a mean and standard deviation. Binary variables (e.g. prevalence, risk) can be analysed using logistic regression with results presented as an odds ratio. While this is frequently used, it must be remembered that this is only valid for rare outcomes, where the prevalence or risk ratio is approximately equal to the odds (see pp. 42–4). Incidence rates may be analysed using other regression models (i.e. Poisson, negative binomial) with results presented as an incidence rate ratio.

If an exposure variable has more than two categories (e.g. ethnicity), we would need to decide which to use as the **reference category** for other categories to be compared against. For example, for a variable with implied ranking such as exposure to smoking, non-smokers may be used as the reference or unexposed group and other categories (e.g. ex-smokers, infrequent smokers, frequent smokers) can each be treated in turn as the exposed group. For a variable such as religion, the choice of reference category is arbitrary. A categorical exposure will result in several relative risks and you will see the relative risk for the reference category presented as 1.00 (i.e. frequency in exposed divided by frequency in unexposed). Differences between non-reference categories can be assessed by comparing their 95% confidence intervals: if they overlap, then there is no significant difference at the $P = 0.05$ level. If the exposure can be quantified (e.g. low, medium or high alcohol consumption), the relative risks can be examined for a dose–response effect.

Regression methods that analyse the effect of just one explanatory variable are called univariate regression models and univariate measures of association are called 'crude' or 'unadjusted'. The real benefit of regression is that we can develop models to look at the effect of multiple variables at the same time, and adjust for potential confounders (see Chapter 4). The resulting measures of association from multivariate regression are 'adjusted' for all the variables included in the model.

Activity 5.5

A study investigated the association between diabetes and the incidence of tuberculosis (TB) in a cohort of individuals. Data were collected on other risk factors for TB, including age, ethnicity, alcohol intake, and smoking.

Table 5.1 Univariate and multivariate incidence rate ratio (IRR) of TB with various risk factors

Variable	Crude IRR (95% CI)	Adjusted IRR (95% CI)
Diabetes:		
No	1	1
Yes	1.20 (1.02–1.41)	1.30 (1.01–1.66)
Smoking:		
Non-smoker	1	1
Ex-smoker	1.23 (1.06–1.44)	1.27 (1.00–1.61)
Current smoker	1.73 (1.48–2.03)	1.67 (1.27–2.19)
Alcohol intake:		
Non-drinker	1	1
Ex-drinker	0.64 (0.44–0.94)	1.00 (0.58–1.73)
Moderate drinker	0.50 (0.42–0.59)	0.86 (0.65–1.13)
Heavy drinker	0.66 (0.51–0.85)	1.04 (0.69–1.59)

Source: Selected data from Pealing et al. (2015).

Table 5.1 shows selected results of the univariate regression (crude) and of the multivariate regression, which adjusts for several variables (not shown here). Interpret the results shown, focusing on the differences between the crude and adjusted estimates for the association between TB and:

1. Diabetes
2. Smoking behaviour
3. Alcohol intake.

Meta-analysis

When several studies of the same exposure–outcome association are available, it may be possible to obtain a combined estimate effect. A *meta-analysis* uses complex statistical techniques to estimate a combined effect from several studies on the assumption that, despite study differences, the increased statistical power will provide an estimate closer to the true value. A systematic literature review is conducted to identify all published and unpublished records of relevant studies. Predefined inclusion and exclusion criteria are used to select studies of sufficiently good quality and where the methodological differences are not too extreme. The measure of association within each study is based on exposed and unexposed groups that are comparable – because comparisons of frequencies across studies would be subject to biases introduced by any study differences.

In its most simple form, a meta-analysis weights the individual estimates in relation to the sample size of each study. A more complex analysis may include individual-level data, with adjustment for study differences. The results of a meta-analysis are usually presented graphically in a forest plot (see Figure 5.6) showing the spread of estimates of effect from individual studies together with the combined estimate of effect. A meta-analysis may be especially useful when faced with conflicting evidence from different studies.

✎ Activity 5.6

1. Describe the variation seen between studies in Figure 5.6.
2. Describe and interpret the combined result.

Dissemination of results

As epidemiological studies involve the participation of human subjects, there is a duty to disseminate the results of these studies not only to the scientific and public health communities, but also to those individuals and

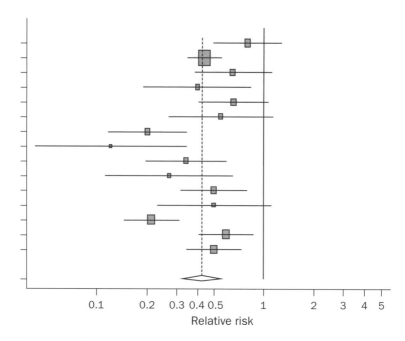

Figure 5.6 Forest plot of estimates from 15 studies of the relative risk of heterosexual HIV infection among circumcised males compared with uncircumcised males

Note: The grey square and horizontal line correspond to the relative risk and 95% CI respectively for each study. The area of the shaded square reflects the weight of each study. The diamond represents the estimate of combined relative risk and 95% confidence interval.

Source: Weiss et al. (2000).

communities participating in the studies. This may be done through leaflets for participants, community meetings, health education campaigns or providing information to support groups (e.g. Parkinson's Disease Society). It may also be appropriate to present the results to ministries of health or local policy-makers and implementers. The dissemination of study findings should be planned from the beginning, as this helps to focus the study on obtaining information that will be relevant to end-users.

Conclusion

In this chapter, you have reviewed the characteristics of the main epidemiological study types and have been introduced to the basics of study design, including sampling, ethics, data collection, analysis, and reporting. These issues should be considered when critically reviewing any epidemiological data and will be discussed further in subsequent chapters.

Feedback on activities in Chapter 5

Feedback on Activity 5.1

1. This is case-control study, with twice as many controls as cases. Study participants were identified in relation to their outcome status, but we were not told how controls were selected. The odds ratio of exposure is the only measure of association that can be calculated for a case-control study.

2. This is a cohort study, which would prospectively measure the incidence of heart disease in relation to various exposures recorded at the start of the study. As this is a follow-up study, the incidence will be measured, so that either the risk ratio or incidence rate ratio (IRR) can be calculated. Given the high likelihood of loss to follow-up for a 10-year study, the most appropriate measure would be the IRR, if person-time at risk has been recorded sufficiently.

3. This is an intervention study, using untreated mosquito nets as the control for an intervention with treated mosquito nets. We are not told if it is a randomized trial or whether observers or participants are blinded to the outcome. The frequency measure is prevalence of anaemia; therefore, the appropriate measure of association would be a prevalence ratio and/or a preventable fraction.

4. This is an ecological study, as the association is measured at a population level. The outcome is national infant mortality and the exposure is gross domestic product, an indicator of standard of living at a population (national) level. The measure of frequency is incidence rate, but because there is no measure of person-time at risk, this is equivalent to a risk. The preferred measure of association would be an IRR.

5. This is a cross-sectional study measuring existing (prevalent) infections, and therefore a prevalence ratio will be the appropriate measure of association.

Feedback on Activity 5.2

1. The outcome measure of interest would be prevalence of males (or females). This is a cluster sample, with all births in a defined period being sampled for each randomly selected district. The inclusion criteria would be all singleton births – that is, multiple births such as twins or triplets would be excluded.

2. The outcome measure of interest would be the prevalence of rubella seropositivity (proportion with rubella antibodies). Simple random sampling was used, as the girls could have been from any of the nine eligible classes. The inclusion criteria would be girls, aged 9–12 years, providing informed (parental) consent (as blood samples would need to be taken).

3. The outcome measure of interest would be access to health care (e.g. percentage of children taken to a health clinic within 48 hours of fever onset). This is a multi-stage sample. First, the regions were selected by simple random sampling and then 5% of households in each region were selected, such that larger regions would contribute more households to the study sample. Inclusion criteria would be households with at least one child under 5 years of age and consenting to participate in the survey.

Feedback on Activity 5.3

1. This is a cross-sectional study (no follow-up) of the relationship between malaria prevalence and household mosquito net ownership. Prevalence is a binary outcome (e.g. Malaria parasites, yes/no), while number of mosquito nets is a quantitative exposure (depending on household size), which could be regrouped as categorical (e.g. 0, 1–2, 3+) or binary (i.e. 0, 1+). The measure of association would be the prevalence ratio. Potential confounders should include socio-economic indicators that are likely to affect both mosquito net ownership and prevalence of malaria (e.g. household wealth, education of household head, house construction materials).

2. This is an occupational cohort study measuring the relationship between employment grade and incidence of all-cause death. The exposure is categorical, and the outcome could be binary (risk of death) or continuous (mortality rate, if the individual person-time at risk is known). The measure of association would be a risk ratio or incidence rate ratio. Likely measurable confounders include age, smoking history, medical conditions, blood pressure, and body mass index (weight divided by height-squared).

3. This is a cohort study following up participants to measure the effect of prescribing practices. The outcome is reported 'risk' of cure after 15 days, which is binary. The explanatory variable is categorical (i.e. number of guideline points met), and it was measured using participant observation. It could be coded as binary (e.g. per guidelines, not per guidelines) or maintained as categorical. The measure of association would be a risk ratio. (Presumably many more than 10 patient consultations would need to be observed to avoid observer influence and to recruit 10 patients with respiratory tract infections.) Confounders would relate to differences between the prescribing doctors and their practices that might also affect outcome. For example, a more conscientious doctor who might prescribe correctly might also be more likely to explain medication instructions, antibiotic compliance, and second-line measures to the patient. Likewise, a busy doctor in an under-resourced neighbourhood may make more prescribing mistakes and the patients may have poorer general health.

4. This is a *matched* case-control study, where each breast cancer case is individually matched with a control. The outcome is binomial (cancer or no cancer), and the explanatory variable may be binomial (previous oral contraceptive use versus none), continuous (number of years of use) or categorical (e.g. none, <2 years, 2–5 years, 5–10 years, 10+ years of oral contraceptive use). The measure of association will be the odds ratio of exposure, as this is a case-control study. Age, many genetic factors, some socio-behavioural factors, family history of breast cancer, and ethnicity have already been controlled for. Potential confounders that may be associated with length of contraceptive use and risk of breast cancer include parity (i.e. number of times a woman has given birth), breast-feeding practices, alcohol consumption, onset of menopause, and physical activity.

Feedback on Activity 5.4

1. This is an ecological study, because the analysis is at a group (national) level.
2. The exposure is national alcohol consumption reported as calories per capita per day, which is a continuous variable. The outcome is incidence of breast cancer per 100,000 person-years, which is also a continuous variable. We can tell that these are continuous variables because they can be presented on a scatterplot.
3. The national incidence of breast cancer appears to increase with increasing national alcohol consumption. However, this is an ecological analysis and we do not know whether this relationship would hold at an individual level.

Feedback on Activity 5.5

1. In the univariate analysis, individuals with diabetes had a 20% increased incidence of TB compared with those without diabetes. However, the lower 95% confidence limit was very close to 1, suggesting that this would be of borderline statistical significance. After adjusting for other variables, individuals with diabetes had a 30% increased incidence of TB, although again this appeared to be of borderline statistical significance.
2. Both the univariate and multivariate analyses appeared to be similar, suggesting that the effect of smoking behaviour on the incidence of TB is not confounded by other variables. The adjusted incidence of TB was 27% greater in ex-smokers compared with non-smokers, although this appeared to be of borderline statistical significance. The adjusted incidence of TB was 67% greater in current smokers compared with non-smokers.
3. In the univariate analysis, alcohol intake appears to be protective, with a reduced incidence rate ratio (IRR) of TB in all categories of alcohol

intake compared with non-drinkers. The effect appears to be statistically significant, as none of the confidence intervals (CIs) overlaps with 1.00. However, after adjusting for other variables, the IRRs are closer to 1 and the CIs overlap with 1.00 for all categories. The comparison of crude and adjusted IRRs suggests that the association between alcohol and TB is confounded by other variables that have been adjusted for in the multivariable model.

Feedback on Activity 5.6

1. Figure 5.6 shows the effect of male circumcision on the risk of hetero-sexual HIV infection in 15 different studies. The forest plot shows that, while there was much variation in estimates between studies, all of them consistently had a relative risk below 1, and this was likely to be statistically significant at the $P < 0.05$ level in 10 of the studies whose CIs did not include 1. As expected, the studies with larger sample sizes (larger shaded squares) had narrower CIs, while those with the smaller sample sizes had wider CIs.

2. The diamond at the bottom of the figure represents the combined result of these 15 studies. This indicates a relative risk of about 0.43 (given by the central point) and a 95% CI of approximately 0.33–0.55 (given by the extremes of the diamond). This suggests that circumcised males have less than 50% risk of heterosexual HIV infection compared with non-circumcised males, or that male circumcision provides approxi-mately 57% protection against infection. The combined result overlaps that of the largest study.

Descriptive epidemiology | 6

Overview

Descriptive epidemiology aims to measure the frequency of health outcomes and their distribution by population, geography, and/or over time. This chapter reviews the different sources of descriptive data, both routine data and data from research studies. You will be introduced to methods for standardizing outcome frequencies to compare data from populations with different demographic structures. The chapter will also consider the use of descriptive epidemiology in investigating outbreaks and emerging health threats.

Learning objectives

When you have completed this chapter, you should be able to:

- review the uses of descriptive epidemiology for research and surveillance
- identify different routine and specialized data sources that may be used
- apply direct and indirect methods of standardization to compare populations
- describe the case distribution and common patterns of outbreaks

Describing health

As you saw in Chapter 1, epidemiology is the study of the distribution and determinants of health. The first step in epidemiology is to *describe* the distribution of a health outcome by measuring its frequency (see Chapter 2) among different individuals or subgroups, across geographic areas, and over time. To understand the extent of a health issue, we need to identify *who* is affected, *where*, and *when*. In addition to highlighting where health resources should be focused, description can identify patterns or anomalies that may indicate a cause. Descriptive epidemiology may use routinely collected data or specially designed studies (Figure 6.1).

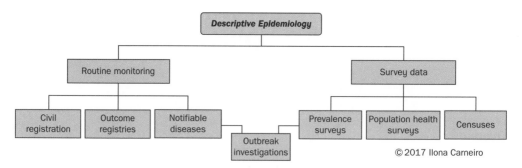

Figure 6.1 Uses of descriptive epidemiology and sources of data

Person

There are many characteristics that may affect an individual's risk of an outcome. These may be biological (e.g. sex, genetics), social (e.g. gender, ethnicity) or behavioural (e.g. exercise, smoking), and some may change over time (e.g. age, diet). In descriptive epidemiology, it is rarely useful to collect data on the frequency of an outcome without collecting additional data on who is affected, to help us understand what we are measuring. Epidemiological data should always include information on age and sex or gender. Where feasible, data collection should include options for intersex, transgender, and/or other locally relevant identities, although numbers for some groups may not be sufficient to present or analyse.

Almost every health outcome is likely to vary with age. For example, there may be a delay in disease progression for chronic outcomes, prior experience for psychiatric outcomes, or variation in exposure by age. For infectious diseases, immunity will be a key factor as age is closely correlated with the development of our immune systems. A cross-sectional survey can provide data on the prevalence of an outcome to describe the health situation and identify which individuals bear the greatest burden (Figure 6.2).

✎ **Activity 6.1**

Describe what Figure 6.2 shows about the prevalence of HIV by age and sex.

Sex (i.e. biological and reproductive characteristics) and/or gender (i.e. social and cultural roles) differences may affect health outcomes. Differences in HIV infection rates between men and women in many studies can partly be explained by gender differences, with younger women tending to have older male partners and women having less ability to negotiate condom use because of a gender-related power imbalance (Krieger, 2003). However,

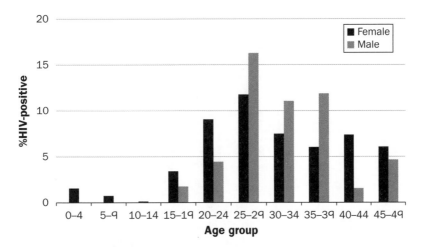

Figure 6.2 HIV-1 prevalence by age and sex in Addis Ababa, Ethiopia, in 1994
Source: Adapted from Fontanet et al. (1998).

there are also biological differences in susceptibility between the sexes, with genital secretions increasing male-to-female HIV transmission and co-infections possibly playing a role.

Place

Climate and other environmental factors can have a marked effect on the distribution of outcomes. For example, insect-borne diseases such as malaria are restricted to tropical and subtropical climates that support mosquito survival for long enough to complete transmission of the parasite between humans or other animal hosts. In Chapter 1, we saw how living upstream or downstream from contaminated water affected residents' risk of cholera, which was incorrectly interpreted by William Farr as being due to elevation.

Data on different geographic areas within a country, and urban or rural residence, may be plotted to enable inequalities in health outcomes and the use of health care to be investigated. The use of geographical information systems enables data to be mapped increasingly precisely, highlighting areas for attention. For example, Figure 6.3 shows the prevalence of obesity by county in the USA in 2007, enabling further epidemiological research and preventive health promotion to be targeted at county level.

Time

By looking at the distribution of an outcome over time, we can identify patterns and track changes. However, if the outcome has a long or unknown **latent** period (i.e. where it is present but not yet detected), time-trend analysis may be more difficult to interpret. Changes in outcome frequency

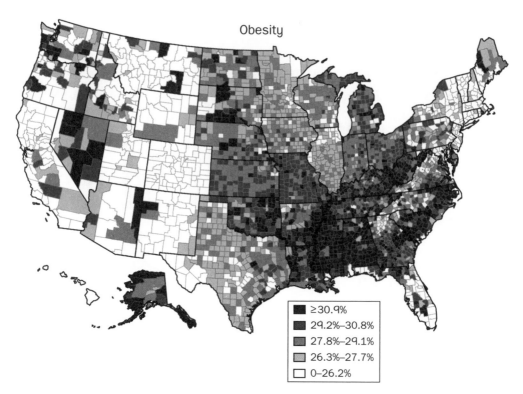

Figure 6.3 Age-adjusted percentage of adults aged ≥20 years who were obese in the USA in 2007
Source: Centers for Disease Control and Prevention (2009).

over time may be described as seasonal or secular. Data can also be used to identify recurrent patterns that may be used to improve health services.

Seasonal trends in frequency refer to changes that occur periodically, usually with a defined time cycle. For example, many childhood infections to which immunity is acquired show cycles of 2–3 years in length. Several outcomes show a seasonal (i.e. intra-annual) pattern that may relate to variations in environment and behaviour. Changes in weather (e.g. temperature, humidity, rain, winds) may affect the survival and spread of a pathogen (e.g. meningitis) or vector (e.g. mosquitoes), and the susceptibility of individuals through altered diet or exposure to sunlight. People also change their behaviour with the season, and increased crowding during colder months will favour transmission of infectious diseases. Once baseline and normal variations are known, unusual changes can be more easily detected, highlighting an **outbreak** or the emergence of a new health problem.

Secular trends refer to changes expected to be sustained over a long period. Changes in time can indicate that public health efforts are working, or alert the health system to a growing health danger. For example, Figure 6.4 shows a decline in syphilis among men and women in the USA between 1996 and 2000, but a concerning increase among men since 2000. As this

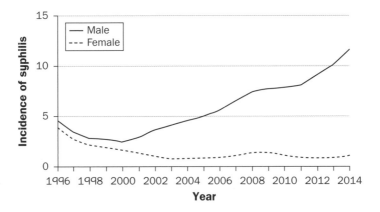

Figure 6.4 Incidence of notified syphilis cases in the USA per 100,000 population per year for males and females

Source: Drawn using data from Centers for Disease Control and Prevention (2009).

is a sexually transmitted disease, the gender disparity over many years suggests that control efforts should be targeted at men who have sex with men.

Secular trends are useful in public health surveillance and planning (see Chapter 10). However, observed changes over time may be related to a modification in the way data are collected or in the case definition. An expansion of the case definition for AIDS in the USA in 1993 led to an artificial increase in the numbers of cases. Changes may also be affected by awareness – for example, an examining doctor may be more likely to diagnose an outcome of interest after a real or suspected outbreak. This can lead to *case-ascertainment bias* (a form of information bias) and an apparent increase in incidence. Such changes need to be documented and alternative explanations considered when interpreting a change in the expected incidence of an outcome.

Activity 6.2

A review was undertaken of deaths within 30 days of elective surgery in hospitals in England (2008–2011). Describe what Table 6.1 shows about mortality in relation to the day on which the procedure was conducted.

Table 6.1 Thirty-day mortality rates (per 1000 admissions) by day of procedure

Surgical procedure	Monday	Tuesday	Wednesday	Thursday	Friday	Weekend
All procedures	5.5	6.2	6.7	7.0	8.2	7.4
Lower-risk procedures	1.8	1.9	2.2	2.2	2.4	1.7

Source: Selected data from Aylin et al. (2013).

Routine data sources

Routinely collected data can provide demographic information (e.g. age, sex, ethnicity) to define a population and describe its overall health through indicators (e.g. birth, fertility, death rates). Data on vital events (e.g. births, deaths) is collected through civil registration systems, censuses, and population health surveys. More specific health outcome data may be collected routinely through health facility data, disease registries, notifiable disease or adverse event reports, population health surveys, and rapid evaluation surveys. However, the accuracy of data depends on the infrastructure available to collect it and how it is used. The more often a data source is used and results fed back to those collecting the information, the greater the incentive to ensure that data are complete, valid, and accurate.

Civil registration

Civil registration systems are used in some countries to collect data on all vital events in the population through legally required official birth and death certification. This provides data on population denominators, demographic structure, birth and mortality rates, and key health indicators. Registration of births may include information on health-related conditions, such as length of gestation, birthweight, and congenital malformations. Mortality data can be used as an indicator of the incidence of specific outcomes, and of the population's overall health. Such data can be used for planning health services, and may be compared between populations and monitored over time to identify issues of concern.

However, the proportion of births and deaths that are registered in a population will be lower in settings with weaker infrastructure for certification and collation of data. The 'completeness' of mortality data (e.g. by cause) will depend on access to formal health services, and is likely to be less in low-income countries and rural areas. Some countries use *sample vital registration* to collect vital data in a nationally **representative sample** of population clusters, which can then be extrapolated to national level. In some countries, demographic surveillance sites collect vital registration data on a defined population, usually for research purposes. While these may not be nationally representative, they may provide useful indications of trends over time.

Censuses

A census is the systematic collection of demographic data about all members of a population (as opposed to a sample), at one time, using a cross-sectional survey design. In countries with inadequate civil registration, data on fertility, mortality, and key health indicators may be estimated from population censuses. These data are useful to assist the planning and allocation of health service resources and policy-making, as they are collected by geographic area. Rigorous methods and quality control are necessary to avoid information bias (e.g. exaggeration of sub-national population if participants perceive that government services will be linked to population size). There will be some *selection bias*, as population subgroups (e.g. homeless, migrant workers) will be under-represented.

In high-income countries, censuses may take the form of postal questionnaires, but countries without sufficient infrastructure require census staff to undertake door-to-door visits. A full population census is ideally carried out at regular intervals (e.g. every 10 years). However, given its complexity and cost, this is not always possible. Statistical methods are used to estimate the data for the intervening years between census surveys, and to make projections about future trends.

Population health indicators

National and sub-national health indicators are commonly presented as incidence rates (e.g. number of live births per 1000 population per year). They can be calculated as epidemiological risks using a fixed population denominator over a defined period, usually one year (see Chapter 2). The information on the population at risk is usually obtained from civil registration or census data. Since population sizes are large, and the outcomes sufficiently rare, relatively small changes in the size of a stable dynamic population should not greatly affect the frequency being measured, and the risk will approximate the rate. Common health indicators presented include neonatal (first 28 days of life), infant (<12 months of age), under 5 (<5 years of age), and maternal mortality per 1000 or 100,000 live births per year.

✎ Activity 6.3

Table 6.2 shows the number of live births, and infant and neonatal deaths, for selected groups of mothers.

1. Calculate the infant and neonatal mortality rates by maternal origin and race/ethnicity.
2. Calculate the percentage of infant deaths that occur under 1 month of age, by maternal race/ethnicity.
3. Compare the infant and neonatal mortality rates between the different maternal categories, and describe the differences.

Table 6.2 Number of live births, and infant and neonatal deaths, for selected groups of maternal origin and race in the USA in 2013

Race/ethnicity of mother	Live births	Infant deaths	Neonatal deaths
Non-Hispanic white	2,129,196	10,766	7119
Non-Hispanic black	583,834	6488	4355
Hispanic	901,033	4507	1911

Source: Selected data from Matthews et al. (2015).

Cause-specific mortality statistics are usually based on identifying a single underlying (primary) cause of death, defined by the WHO as the 'disease or injury that initiated the series of events leading directly to death, or the circumstances of the accident or violence that produced the fatal injury'. In settings where many individuals do not access formal health services, a verbal autopsy method may be used for a sample of the population. This involves a structured interview with family members to understand the circumstances surrounding the death and classify its cause. Additional data are recorded on significant conditions or diseases (e.g. diabetes) that may have contributed to the death.

A single standardized coding system is used when death certificates are collated, allowing the comparison of mortality within countries, over time, and with other countries. Trained personnel use the International Classification of Diseases (ICD), the tenth version of which came into use in 1994, to code cause of death. However, there may be *information bias* related to the accuracy of clinical diagnoses, completion of death registration or subsequent coding. For example, outcomes that are stigmatized (e.g. maternal death due to illegal abortion, suicide, HIV/AIDS) may not be accurately reported. Such factors need to be considered when using and interpreting these data.

Outcome-specific data

In settings with robust infrastructure, routine data from health facilities may prove useful. For example, hospital admissions, clinic attendance, and laboratory results may provide sufficient information to describe the health of the local population, or identify the appearance of a new problem. At a national or sub-national level, outcome-specific data may be collated for surveillance purposes. These sources of surveillance data are discussed further in Chapter 10.

Patient registries involve the systematic collection of data about every patient with a specific diagnosis, condition or procedure (e.g. cancer, artificial joints). **Notifiable diseases** (e.g. yellow fever) require compulsory (i.e. legally enforced) reporting, while voluntary reporting systems include adverse reactions to medications by physicians and patients (e.g. the Adverse Event Reporting System in the USA). Sentinel surveillance through networks of health facilities or laboratories may also provide quality-controlled systems, for example to detect cases of polio or the spread of antimicrobial resistance.

Cross-sectional surveys

When routine data are non-existent, unreliable or insufficient for research needs, a more tailor-made approach to data collection is required. Rapid assessment of large numbers of individuals at one point in time can be undertaken for situation analysis using cross-sectional surveys. These are sometimes called 'prevalence surveys', as they measure the frequency of an existing outcome or exposure, and may provide a baseline for further monitoring or research. Surveys provide a snapshot of a population's current health status and can be used to indicate the extent of a health problem, identify health service needs, determine lifestyle practices, generate hypotheses, and design analytical epidemiological studies. Cross-sectional surveys may be designed to collect information on specific subgroups (e.g. migrants, those not accessing routine services) or to assess the effect of an intervention (e.g. cluster sampling to assess vaccination coverage after a measles campaign).

Population health surveys

Cross-sectional population health surveys are conducted in countries with unreliable or insufficient routine data, to provide information on population health indicators (see above) using a representative sample of the population. Repeated surveys can be used to determine changes over time and often form a core part of monitoring. The Demographic and Health Survey (DHS) Program collects and disseminates nationally representative data from household surveys in low- and middle-income countries using standardized data collection and analysis methods (https://dhsprogram.com/). UNICEF undertakes Multiple Indicator Cluster Surveys to provide information on selected women's and children's health indicators (http://www.mics.unicef.org/). Another example is the National Health and Nutrition Examination Survey (NHANES), which is used to assess health and nutritional status in the USA through a combination of interviews and physical examinations (https://www.cdc.gov/nchs/nhanes/).

Study design

A representative sample is selected using random selection and sample size calculation methods discussed in Chapter 5. A **pilot study** is often undertaken to pre-test data collection and data entry methods, and to reduce errors or identify possible problems. Appropriate design and training can help to limit mistakes when completing questionnaires and improve response rates to difficult questions. However, if difficulties are anticipated (e.g. respondents may refuse to answer sensitive questions on income or sexual behaviours, or if infants may not release enough blood for a finger-prick sample), this can be accounted for by increasing the sample size in advance.

Cross-sectional studies may collect information using a combination of questionnaires and diagnostic tests. Although data are collected at one time point, the measures collected may be current (e.g. blood pressure, current symptoms) or past (e.g. vaccination history, previous smoking practices). It is important that survey questions are sufficiently specific. For example, asking 'Did your child have fever in the last 24 hours?' will provide an estimate of the point prevalence of (current) fever. However, asking 'Has your child had fever during the last 2 weeks?' will record fever episodes that started prior to 2 weeks and continued into it, as well as episodes that started during the 2-week period of interest, making the answers difficult to interpret. Surveys that relate to the prevalence of an outcome during a period in the past will estimate period prevalence. While period prevalence may increase case detection and therefore reduce the necessary sample size, questions about prior experience may also increase the possibility of *recall bias*.

Questions need to be appropriately designed and tested to improve response rates. A question that is unclear, or that the respondent may be embarrassed to answer, can result in non-responder bias (a form of information bias). Choosing appropriate methods for the topic of investigation (e.g. interview vs self-completed questionnaire), ensuring confidentiality and anonymity, and careful wording and pre-testing of questions should reduce such error.

✎ Activity 6.4

Published data from the National Health and Nutrition Survey in Japan were used to examine changes in the consumption of different food groups over time. Annual cross-sectional surveys included clinical and laboratory assessment, dietary assessment, and a questionnaire on dietary and lifestyle habits. Figure 6.5 presents the differences in food intake from the 1999 and 2009 surveys, compared with the 1989 survey results.

1. Describe the differences for each food category over time, and compare the results for males and females.
2. From the information provided, identify possible limitations of this study.

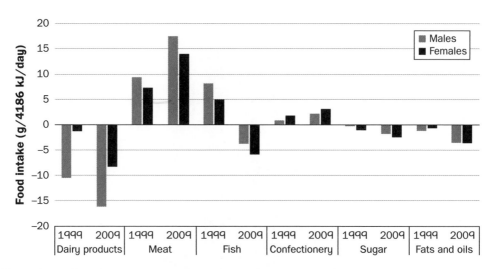

Figure 6.5 Differences in mean adult food intake by gender in 1999 and 2009 compared with 1989 survey results from national surveys in Japan

Source: Drawn using data from Otsuka et al. (2014).

Standardization

Descriptive data may come from different places (e.g. countries, regions within a country) or from the same population during different time periods. Comparing the 'crude' or overall incidence rate of an outcome across populations or time periods may be inaccurate due to differences between these populations in factors that are known to modify or confound the outcome (e.g. age, tobacco exposure).

For example, Figure 6.6 shows that the population of South Africa consists of many children and young adults, whereas Switzerland has an older population. What effect does this have if we want to compare cancer mortality rates between these countries? The mortality rate for all cancers in males in 2013 was 229 per 100,000 in Switzerland and 71 per 100,000 in South Africa (World Health Organization, 2016b). If we calculate the incidence rate ratio (229 ÷ 71 = 3.23), we may conclude that males living in Switzerland have a three times greater risk of dying from cancer than those living in South Africa. However, if we look at age-specific cancer mortality rates, we see that they are similar for both countries until the oldest age group (Figure 6.7), suggesting that the difference in crude rates is due to the different age distributions.

To compare the data properly, we need to find the overall frequency expected if these populations had the same age distribution. This is known as **standardization**, where the structure (relative distribution) of two populations is equalized with respect to an outcome-modifying factor, enabling their comparison to be 'standardized' for that factor. There are two methods

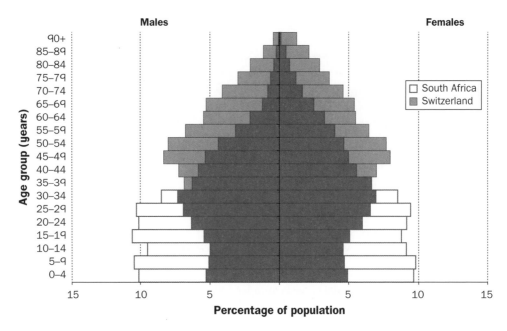

Figure 6.6 Estimated population age distribution of males and females in South Africa and Switzerland in 2015

Source: Drawn using data from United Nations (2015b).

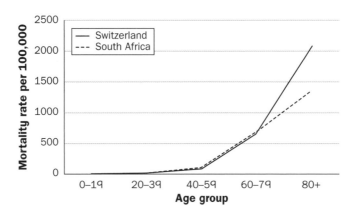

Figure 6.7 Age-specific male cancer mortality rates in 2013 for Switzerland and South Africa

Source: Drawn using data from United Nations (2015b) and World Health Organization (2016b).

of standardization: one enables a *direct* comparison of standardized outcome frequencies (prevalence or incidence) in different populations; the other enables an *indirect* comparison through calculation of a standardized ratio of the frequency difference between populations.

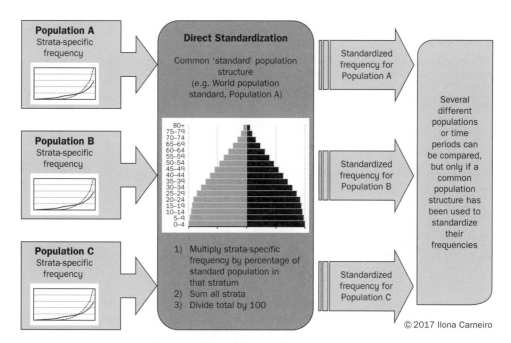

Figure 6.8 Schematic of direct standardization, showing the sources of data and methodology used

Direct standardization

Direct standardization is used when we know the strata-specific outcome frequency (i.e. number of cases divided by the total number at risk in each subgroup) in the populations we are comparing (Figure 6.8). These frequencies are applied to a common population structure, called the **standard population**, to calculate a weighted-average frequency for each comparison population, called a **standardized frequency**. A standardized frequency cannot be used as a real value, because it does not relate to a real population, time, and place, but allows us to better compare populations.

Age standardization is most commonly undertaken, and will be described here, although the same methods can be applied to standardization for other outcome-modifying factors (e.g. gender, socio-economic status). Data on the population age structure may be available from a census or vital registration data. There are also recognized 'standards'; for example, the World Standard Population developed by the WHO is based on the predicted average age structure of the world's population from 2000 to 2025 (Ahmad et al., 2001). However, it does not matter which standard is used, so long as the same population structure is used for all populations being compared.

Table 6.3 shows the age-specific mortality rates that underlie Figure 6.7. To undertake direct standardization, we multiply the percentage of the

Table 6.3 Direct standardization of Swiss and South African (SA) male cancer mortality rates per 100,000 in 2013

Age group (years)	World Standard Population (%)	Swiss age-specific mortality rate*	Swiss weighted mortality measure	SA age-specific mortality rate*
0–19	34.61	2.35	81.33	2.59
20–39	30.90	8.55	264.20	13.34
40–59	22.54	89.63	2020.26	115.69
60–79	10.41	654.11	6809.29	694.63
85+	1.54	2071.26	3189.74	1355.68
Total	100.00		12,364.81	

* Per 100,000 population.

Source: Data from Ahmad et al. (2001), United Nations (2015b), and World Health Organization (2016b).

standard population for each age group (Column 2) by the mortality rate in our population of interest (Column 3) for that age group. The sum of these weighted measures across all age groups (Column 4) gives a total weighted average mortality, which we divide by 100 to get an age-standardized cancer mortality rate of 124 per 100,000 for Swiss males in 2013.

 Activity 6.5

1. Calculate an age-standardized cancer mortality rate for South African males using Table 6.3.
2. Compare the age-standardized rate of male cancer mortality in South Africa with that of 124 per 100,000 in Switzerland in 2013, and interpret these findings.

Indirect standardization

Indirect standardization is used when we don't have strata-specific frequency data for our population of interest, but we know the population structure and the total number of cases. Strata-specific frequencies from a comparison population are applied to our population of interest, to calculate the total number of cases expected if they had the same structure (Figure 6.9).

The expected number of cases is then used to calculate a **standardized ratio** (SR), which compares the observed outcome frequency with expected frequency. This is usually calculated for mortality rates and is best known

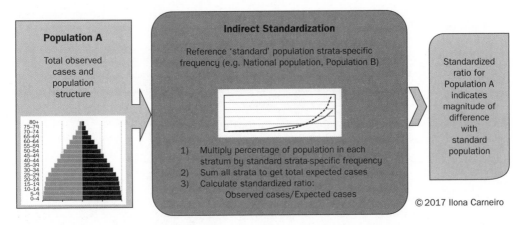

Figure 6.9 Schematic of indirect standardization, showing the sources of data and methodology used

as the standardized mortality rate (SMR), but can also be applied to prevalence, risk or incidence rate. It is calculated as:

$$\text{Standardized ratio} = \frac{\text{Observed cases}}{\text{Expected cases}}$$

A standardized ratio is interpreted in the same way as a relative risk, comparing the study population to a reference 'standard' population. As the indirect standardization method does not use a common standard age structure, SRs calculated for several different populations should not be compared with each other, unless the population structures are shown to be comparable.

✎ Activity 6.6

There were 35,471 reported cancer deaths among males in Mexico in 2013. The estimated age distribution for males in Mexico in 2015 is given in Table 6.4. Using the data provided:

1. Estimate the crude cancer mortality rate for males in Mexico, and calculate an incidence rate ratio to compare it with the estimate of 229 per 100,000 for Switzerland.
2. Fill in the last column of Table 6.4 (note the units), calculate a standardized mortality ratio for Mexico compared with Switzerland, and interpret the result.

Table 6.4 Age distribution for males in Mexico and age-specific cancer mortality rate among males in Switzerland

Age group (years)	Mexico male population (1000s)	Swiss male cancer mortality rate (per 100,000 population)	Expected cancer cases among males in Mexico
0–19	23,943	2.35	563
20–39	20,534	8.55	
40–59	13,009	89.63	
60–79	4925	654.11	
85+	770	2071.26	

Source: Data from United Nations (2015b) and World Health Organization (2016b).

Outbreak investigations

Another use of descriptive epidemiology involves the detection of new health risks (several cases of an outcome not previously seen in the population), clusters (an aggregation of cases geographically or over time) or disease outbreaks (the occurrence of more cases than expected). An outbreak may be referred to as an **epidemic** when it has a wider geographical distribution and as a **pandemic** when it spreads across populations and countries. Expected seasonal variation must be incorporated into any estimates of baseline incidence to distinguish seasonal peaks from the start of an outbreak. An increase in cases may be identified through a review of routine data, or through reports of cases by clinicians, laboratories or members of the public. For example, at the start of the AIDS epidemic, clinicians presented several unusual case reports with similar features. If the severity of the outcome or the number of cases is of sufficient concern, further investigation should be undertaken.

Once a problem is suspected, a rapid situation analysis is necessary to identify the extent of the problem. Data must be collected and analysed on those at risk and potential risk factors. As with all epidemiological studies, the first step is to have a clear definition of what is to be measured. In the early stages of describing a new health outcome, the case definition may be less specific to ensure that cases are not missed. It is always possible to narrow the definition later and exclude non-cases when more information is available, but not always possible to identify cases that have been missed. It is also important not to include any factors in this case definition that may be related to a possible cause or risk factor, as this could prevent detection of all cases and reduce evidence for causality.

Case ascertainment

Additional cases may be identified through clinicians or health facilities, or by notifying the public and appealing for people to come forward with information. Case ascertainment methods will vary with the outcome and the health infrastructure of the setting, but may be passive or active. **Passive surveillance** means that cases are detected when they seek help. Investigators can contact health service providers (e.g. clinicians, laboratories, health centres) to ask for reports of new cases meeting the definition, or to ask them to review their records to identify possible cases retrospectively.

If a sufficient proportion of those affected might not access formal health care, the health infrastructure is weak or the situation is urgent, investigators can use **active surveillance**. This may involve a cross-sectional survey to identify prevalent cases, for example if the outbreak is restricted to a hospital or school, or if there are likely to be many asymptomatic cases that would not otherwise be detected. Depending on the case definition, a survey could involve a questionnaire about symptoms, a clinical examination, and/or samples for laboratory analyses. Cases may also be able to identify others with the same condition, and *contact tracing* can be used for infectious diseases, identifying people who may have had contact with a case, for testing or further surveillance. This is especially important to stop the spread of highly infectious diseases (e.g. Ebola), and is often used for sexually transmitted infections (e.g. HIV, chlamydia).

Outbreak description

Once the data are collated, they can be summarized to identify the people and places at risk, and to visualize any trends over time. By looking at the data early, we can identify our knowledge gaps and determine what data or studies are required to better describe the outcome. A histogram plot of the number of cases by time, or 'epidemic curve', is a simple way to visualize the problem. We ideally want to know the reported time or date of onset of each case, rather than when it was detected, as this can vary considerably between cases.

Typical patterns of epidemic curves are shown in Figure 6.10, and with sufficient data they can help us to identify the type of exposure and mode of transmission. A steep rise in cases followed by a gradual decline indicates exposure to a common source. A common source of cases may occur at one point (e.g. food poisoning), intermittently (e.g. sporadic release of toxic waste) or continuously (e.g. undetected water contamination). A propagated epidemic indicates an infectious agent being spread successively through a population, and although it may initially show distinct epidemic peaks, which may increase in size, these will eventually

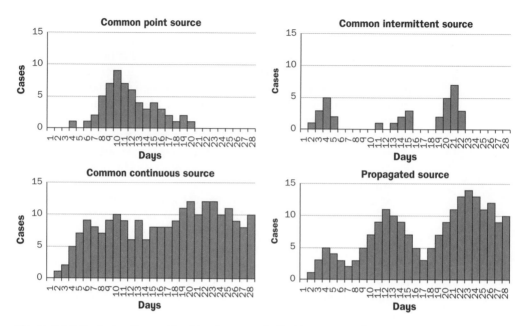

Figure 6.10 Typical patterns of epidemic curves indicating source of exposure and transmission

merge. Without information on the incubation period of an outcome, it may be difficult to distinguish between different patterns. Some outcomes, such as vector-borne diseases, are likely to show a similar pattern to a continuous source epidemic, and other outbreaks may follow a mixture or none of the patterns in Figure 6.10.

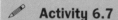 **Activity 6.7**

Figure 6.11 shows the distribution of suspected, probable, and confirmed cases of Ebola virus disease (EVD) in the Democratic Republic of Congo (DRC) outbreak of 26 July to 4 October 2014. Referring to the probable and confirmed cases combined:

1. Describe the age distribution of EVD in this outbreak.
2. Identify the type of epidemic curve, and suggest what this may indicate about the source of the outbreak.

Identifying the causes of an outbreak will require analytical epidemiological methods, which are discussed in subsequent chapters, while routine surveillance and outbreak responses are discussed in Chapter 10.

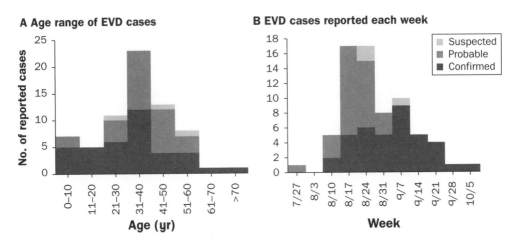

Figure 6.11 Cases of Ebola virus disease (EVD) in the Democratic Republic of Congo in 2014 by age (A) and weekly incidence (B)

Source: Maganga et al. (2014).

Conclusion

In this chapter, we have reviewed sources of routine and specific data for descriptive epidemiology. You should now be able to describe how measures of frequency, and their distribution by population, place, and time, can be used to gain a better understanding of the burden of health outcomes and to identify healthcare needs.

Additional activities to test your understanding

 Activity 6.8

Road traffic mortality rates for two European countries were reported for 2015 as 1689/46,122,000 for Country X and 3459/80,689,000 for Country Y.

1. Compare the crude road traffic mortality rates for Countries X and Y in 2015.
2. Use Table 6.5 to calculate an age-standardized measure of comparison between these two road traffic mortality rates for 2015. Interpret your result.

Table 6.5 Country X population age distribution and road traffic mortality rates by age for Countries X and Y in 2015

Age group (years)	Population of Country X (%)	Country X age-specific mortality rate*	Country Y age-specific mortality rate*
<17	17.6	0.64	1.22
18–24	5.7	5.48	9.30
25–49	36.9	3.87	4.01
50–64	21.0	3.30	3.85
65+	18.8	5.82	5.99

* Per 100,000 population

 Activity 6.9

The estimated national prevalence of asthma in children under 15 years was 4% and 2% for countries A and B respectively. However, cross-sectional surveys in country A found the prevalence of asthma to be 5% in urban areas and 1.5% in rural areas. The population of country B had an estimated 1 million children aged under 15 years living in urban areas and 3 million living in rural areas.

1. Calculate an epidemiological measure of the crude asthma prevalence in country B compared with country A, and interpret your answer.
2. Calculate a standardized ratio of prevalence to compare the national estimates of asthma after adjusting for differences in the urban/rural population distribution between countries A and B, and interpret your answer.

Feedback on activities in Chapter 6

Feedback on Activity 6.1

Your answer may have included the following: Figure 6.2 shows that the burden of HIV infection is concentrated in adults. As HIV is sexually transmitted, this age distribution corresponds with the sexually active age groups, peaking in the 25–29 year age group. The few cases in young children are probably the result of mother-to-child transmission. Women appear to be infected with HIV at younger ages than men, possibly due to younger sexual debut or older sexual partners.

Feedback on Activity 6.2

The data in Table 6.1 suggest that the 30-day mortality rate increases with day of the week, being highest for procedures on Fridays. For all surgical procedures, 30-day mortality is highest for Friday and weekend procedures. However, for lower-risk surgery, 30-day mortality is lowest for weekend procedures. This may suggest that lower-risk procedures are less likely than higher-risk procedures to be undertaken on weekends. [*Note*: This is a healthcare phenomenon known as the 'weekend effect', in which outcomes are sometimes found to be worse at the weekend.]

Feedback on Activity 6.3

1. Table 6.6 shows the infant and neonatal mortality rates you should have calculated. Infant and neonatal mortality rates are calculated as the number of deaths divided by the number of live births for the same population and period. For example, infant mortality for non-Hispanic white mothers is $10,766 \div 2,129,196 = 0.00506$, or 5.06 per 1000 live births.
2. The last column of Table 6.6 shows the percentage of infant deaths that occur under 1 month of age. It is calculated by dividing the number of neonatal deaths by the number of infant deaths for each subgroup, e.g. $7119 \div 10,766 = 0.66$, or 66%. You may also have divided the rate in Column 2 by that in Column 1 = $3.34 \div 5.06 = 0.66$.

   The infant mortality rate is similar among non-Hispanic white and Hispanic mothers, with non-Hispanic black mothers having a much higher infant mortality. Neonatal mortality is also higher among non-Hispanic black mothers than among other groups. Comparison of neonatal deaths as a percentage of all infant deaths shows that Hispanic mothers appear to have fewer neonatal deaths than non-Hispanic mothers.

Table 6.6 Results for Activity 6.3

Race/ethnicity of mother	Infant mortality rate per 1000 live births	Neonatal mortality rate per 1000 live births	Percentage of infant deaths <1 month (%)
Non-Hispanic white	5.06	3.34	66.12
Non-Hispanic black	11.11	7.46	67.12
Hispanic	5.00	2.12	42.40

Feedback on Activity 6.4

1. These data suggest some secular changes in Japanese diet over time. There appears to be a decrease in consumption of dairy products over time among males, which is less pronounced – or delayed – among females. Both sugar and fats and oils consumption declined over time for both genders. Meat and confectionery consumption increased over time for both genders. Fish consumption increased initially, but then declined for both genders. [*Note*: The lack of any confidence intervals or *P*-values means that comparisons of the magnitudes of change by gender and time are subjective.]
2. You may have mentioned the following possible limitations, among others:

- If consumption information is based on reported intake, it may be subject to recall or reporting biases.
- We are not told how foods are classified or measured. It is possible that changes in measurement or food classification criteria over time may have contributed to some of the effects seen (e.g. the inconsistencies in fish consumption). However, this is unlikely to explain the gender differences seen for dairy intake.
- The presentation of only three surveys may lead to random fluctuations being interpreted as trends. Presentation of data from all annual surveys would provide more information on whether there really are secular trends.

Feedback on Activity 6.5

1. You should have multiplied the SA age-specific mortality rate by the percentage of the World Standard Population for each age group in Table 6.3, to get a weighted measure of mortality for each age group (Table 6.7). The sum of these divided by 100 gives an age-standardized male cancer mortality rate for South Africa of 124 per 100,000.
2. The age-standardized rates are very similar in the two populations, with an incidence rate ratio of 1.00 or 0.99 using un-rounded data. This indicates that after adjusting for differences in age structure, there is no difference in the overall incidence rate of cancer mortality in males in 2013 between Switzerland and South Africa.

Feedback on Activity 6.6

1. We can sum the male population in all strata from Table 6.4 to calculate a total estimated male population in Mexico of 63,181,000 in 2015. The crude cancer mortality rate for males in Mexico is calculated from the total number of cases divided by the total population at risk: 35,471 ÷ 63,181,000 = 56 per 100,000. [*Note*: This will be an underestimate, as

the population in 2013 is likely to have been smaller than in 2015.] This would indicate an incidence rate ratio of $56 \div 229 = 0.24$, suggesting that males in Mexico are 76% less likely to die of cancer than males in Switzerland.

2. The number of expected cases in each age group in Mexico is calculated by multiplying the number of males in each category (in 1000s) by the Swiss age-specific mortality rate divided by 100, because it is per 100,000 population (see Table 6.8). The sum of expected cancer cases among males if Mexico had the same age-specific cancer rates as Switzerland was 62,143. Therefore, the standardized mortality rate (SMR) = observed cases/expected cases = $35,471/62,143 = 0.57$. This suggests that males in Mexico are 43% less likely to die of cancer

Table 6.7 Direct standardization of Swiss and South African (SA) male cancer mortality rates per 100,000 in 2013

Age group (years)	World Standard Population (%)	Swiss age-specific mortality rate*	Swiss weighted mortality measure	SA age-specific mortality rate*	SA weighted mortality measure
0–19	34.61	2.35	81.33	2.59	89.64
20–39	30.90	8.55	264.20	13.34	412.21
40–59	22.54	89.63	2020.26	115.69	2607.65
60–79	10.41	654.11	6809.29	694.63	7231.10
85+	1.54	2071.26	3189.74	1355.68	2087.75
Total	100.00		12,364.81		12,428.34

* Per 100,000 population.

Source: Data from Ahmad et al. (2001), United Nations (2015b), and World Health Organization (2016b).

Table 6.8 Numbers of cancer cases expected by age group in Mexico using the Swiss age-specific rates

Age group (years)	Mexico male population (1000s)	Swiss male cancer mortality rate per 100,000 population	Expected cancer cases among males in Mexico
0–19	23,943	2.35	563
20–39	20,534	8.55	1756
40–59	13,009	89.63	11,660
60–79	4925	654.11	32,215
85+	770	2071.26	15,949
Total	63,181		62,143

than males in Switzerland, after standardizing for differences in the population age distribution. [*Note*: This assumes comparable systems of cancer mortality reporting between the two populations, and stable populations between 2013 and 2015.]

Feedback on Activity 6.7

1. EVD cases were reported in all age groups and peaked in adults (age 21–60 years). Cases were more common in children than in older adults (61+), but these are case numbers and not incidence, so we don't know whether this is just a function of the age distribution of the population at risk.

2. You may have said that the weekly distribution of EVD cases resembles a common point source epidemic curve, where the initial case in the week of 27 July represents the source of the epidemic. Alternatively, you may have thought that the distribution resembles a propagated source with one peak in August and another in September. [*Note*: It is not easy to distinguish between these two from the graph shown. However, our knowledge of Ebola transmission would suggest that this was a propagated source, and this may have been clearer if the data had been available for daily rather than weekly cases.]

Feedback on Activity 6.8

1. The crude road traffic mortality rates were 1689 ÷ 46,122,000 = 3.66 per 100,000 population for Country X and 3459 ÷ 80,689,000 = 4.29 per 100,000 for Country Y in 2015. Calculating a mortality **rate ratio** of 4.29 ÷ 3.66 = 1.17, suggests that there are 17% more road traffic deaths in Country Y compared with Country X.

2. The data in Table 6.5 show variability in age-specific rates, and with rates consistently higher for Country Y than Country X in each age group. As we have age-specific mortality rates, we can use direct standardization to calculate an age-standardized total population rate for each country. Because we have the Country X population structure for 2015, we do not need to do anything with these data, as the 'crude' mortality rate will already be age-standardized to the Country X population in 2015. However, we can calculate the mortality rate for Country Y, age-standardized to the Country X population, as in Table 6.9 by multiplying across columns (e.g. for <17 years: 17.6 × 1.22 = 21.47). We then sum and divide by 100 because we used a percentage age distribution to standardize. This gives us an overall age-standardized rate for Country Y of 4.16 per 100,000. After age standardization, we can calculate a standardized rate ratio of 4.16 ÷ 3.66 = 1.14, suggesting that there are 14% more road traffic deaths in Country Y compared with Country X after adjusting for differences in the age distribution between these countries.

Table 6.9 Age standardization of Country Y road traffic mortality rate

Age group (years)	Population of Country X (%)	Country Y age-specific mortality rate*	Country Y weighted age-specific mortality
<17	17.6	1.22	21.47
18–24	5.7	9.30	53.01
25–49	36.9	4.01	147.97
50–64	21.0	3.85	80.85
65+	18.8	5.99	112.61
Total	100.00		415.91

* Per 100,000 population.

Feedback on Activity 6.9

1. The crude asthma prevalence can be compared by calculating a prevalence ratio = 0.02 ÷ 0.04 = 0.50, indicating that Country B has 50% or half the childhood asthma of Country A. If you calculated this the other way around, you would have obtained a prevalence ratio of 0.04 ÷ 0.02 = 2.00, i.e. double the asthma prevalence in Country A compared with Country B.
2. The data can be indirectly standardized by applying the strata-specific asthma prevalence of Country A to the population of Country B, and summing the cases (Table 6.10). A total of 95,000 childhood asthma cases would be expected in Country B after standardizing. The observed cases would be 2% of the total child population = 0.02 × (1,000,000 + 3,000,000) = 80,000. The standardized prevalence ratio = observed cases divided by expected cases = 80,000 ÷ 95,000 = 0.84. This means that after adjusting for differences in urban and rural population distribution, there would be 0.84 times or 16% fewer cases in Country B compared with Country A. This suggests that most of the difference in childhood asthma prevalence seen between these two countries is due to differences in the urban/rural distribution of their populations.

Table 6.10 Indirect standardization of Country B asthma prevalence by urban and rural population distribution

Residence	Population of children under 15 years in Country B	Country A strata-specific asthma prevalence	Country B strata-specific expected asthma cases
Urban	1,000,000	0.050	50,000
Rural	3,000,000	0.015	45,000
Total			95,000

7 Analytical studies

Overview

Once a health concern has been identified using descriptive epidemiology, we need to conduct further investigations in the form of analytical studies. In this chapter, we review specific issues related to the choice, design, analysis, and interpretation of the key analytical study designs: ecological, cross-sectional, cohort, and case-control. We will review the use of ecological studies for group-level analysis, cross-sectional studies to identify possible epidemiological associations rapidly, cohort studies to follow the natural course of exposure-outcome progression, and case-control studies for new or rare outcomes.

Learning objectives

When you have completed this chapter, you should be able to:

- describe key features of different analytical study designs
- identify appropriate study designs for a given health problem
- discuss sources of potential bias and confounding in different analytical studies
- interpret results from different study designs

Key features of analytical study designs

Analytical investigations are undertaken to detect or confirm hypothesized epidemiological associations. Ecological and cross-sectional studies are relatively cheap and easy to conduct, and are often used to show the existence of an association, and to provide preliminary data for planning further studies. Cohort and case-control studies usually provide better evidence of causality, but are more logistically complex and expensive. However, a simple, well-designed study is better than a complex, poorly designed one.

The choice of which analytical study design to undertake will depend on several factors: existing information available about the association of interest, level at which the exposure acts, expected frequency of the outcome, urgency of identifying the cause (e.g. outbreaks), as well as logistical constraints such as time, budget, and personnel. Each study design has advan-

Table 7.1 Key features, advantages, and disadvantages of main analytical study designs

Study design	Key features	Advantages	Disadvantages
Ecological	Population-based Prevalence of incident cases Group-level effects Measure correlation or any relative risk	Relatively easy to collect data (routine) Rapid Relatively inexpensive	High probability of confounding Medium probability of selection bias Cannot show causality at the individual level ('ecological fallacy')
Cross-sectional	Outcome and exposure measured simultaneously Prevalent cases Measure association as prevalence ratio (or odds ratio if outcome is rare)	Easy to collect data Rapid Inexpensive Good for fixed exposures (e.g. genetic)	High probability of information bias (possibility of 'reverse causality') Medium probability of confounding
Cohort	Exposure determined before cases detected Incident cases Measure association as risk ratio or incidence rate ratio	Low probability of selection bias Low probability of confounding Multiple outcomes	Medium to high probability of loss to follow-up (for long studies) Logistically difficult Expensive Time-consuming
Case-control	Participants selected by outcome; exposure determined subsequently Prevalent cases Measure association as odds ratio of exposure	Can be rapid (good for outbreaks) Relatively inexpensive Efficient for rare outcomes Multiple exposures	High probability of selection and information bias Medium probability of confounding No data on frequency of outcome

tages and disadvantages (see Table 7.1) and several designs may be necessary to accumulate sufficient evidence of causality. We will review the defining features, strengths, and limitations of each analytical design.

Ecological studies

The defining feature of an ecological study is that the association between outcome and exposure is measured at the population level, where 'population' represents a group of individuals with a shared characteristic such as geography, ethnicity, socio-economic status or employment. Data on outcome and exposure may be measured at an individual level and then aggregated at a group level (e.g. census or registry data); they may vary by individual but be measured or estimated at a group level (e.g. maternal mortality rate); or they may be attributes of the group that do not vary by individual (e.g. gross national product).

In ecological studies, measures of exposure and outcome are often continuous (e.g. disease prevalence, mortality rate, proportion of population exposed, mean temperature in a geographical region). Such data are displayed as a scatterplot to identify any relationship in the data, which can then be confirmed using correlation or regression models (see Chapter 5). Alternatively, if the outcome can be categorized into two groups, we can estimate the relative risk of outcome for a given exposure. Regression models can then be used to estimate the relative risk for continuous exposures and/or adjust for potential confounders. As you saw in Chapter 6, it may be necessary to standardize data first, if the groups being compared have different population structures with respect to any modifying factors.

However, ecological studies cannot be used to infer causality at an individual level, because there may be a mismatch between individual- and group-level data. To draw conclusions about individual-level associations from a group-level study is known as an **ecological fallacy**. Consider a study showing a correlation between the prevalence of rhesus-negative individuals (Rh-) and chronic heart disease (CHD): population A has 20% CHD and 20% Rh-, population B has 30% CHD and 30% Rh-, and population C has 50% CHD and 50% Rh-. Figure 7.1 demonstrates how there may be no real association at the individual level, despite an apparent perfect correlation at the population level.

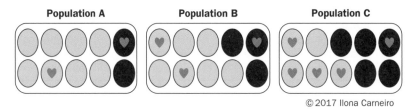

© 2017 Ilona Carneiro

Figure 7.1 Representation of ecological fallacy across three populations

Note: Dark ovals represent rhesus-negative (Rh-) individuals and a heart represents those with chronic heart disease (CHD).

Advantages of ecological studies

The main reasons for undertaking an ecological study are:

- when data are readily available at a group level, as with routine data;
- when the exposure can be measured only at a group level (e.g. air pollution);
- if data are difficult to measure at an individual level because of considerable variation, and group averages may be more consistent (e.g. ethnic or social differences in alcohol consumption); or

- to study group-level effects (e.g. public health interventions through policy or legislation, such as injury prevention through national road safety laws), because individual-level associations may not translate into group-level effects.

As with descriptive studies, an ecological study may compare populations, geographical areas ('spatial patterns'), periods of time ('time-trends'), or groups and time using a 'mixed design'. Routine data are often used for ecological analyses, because they are readily available. The World Health Organization (WHO) publishes estimates of population size and key health indicators for its 194 member states through the Global Health Observatory (World Health Organization, 2017a). While these may not be as detailed as some locally collected data, they use standardized definitions, enabling more valid comparisons. For example, Figure 7.2 shows the association between national gross domestic product and life expectancy for 169 countries.

Ecological studies are often used to compare spatial patterns in the frequency of an outcome. For example, by comparing the geographical distribution of populations with a high frequency of genetic blood disorders (e.g. thalassaemia) with that of malaria, it was suggested that such genes might provide some protection against malaria infection. The use of geographical information systems (see Chapter 5) has enabled more sophisticated analyses of environmental risks for health outcomes.

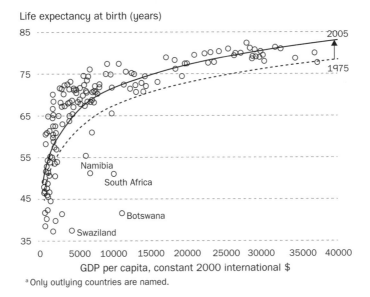

Figure 7.2 Gross domestic product (GDP) per capita and life expectancy at birth in 169 countries (1975 and 2005)

Source: World Health Organization (2008).

Time-trend studies investigate whether changes in the incidence of an outcome over time correlate with changes in risk factors or coverage of an intervention over the same period (e.g. changes in air quality and incidence of asthma in children). However, the association between exposure and outcome may vary over time, making interpretation of a time-trend analysis more complicated. Mixed-studies compare different groups over time and if consistent differences are seen, this may lend weight to a causal association, as in Bradford Hill's considerations for causality (see Chapter 4).

✐ Activity 7.1

An ecological study was conducted to investigate the effect of air pollutants on pregnancy outcomes estimated from routinely collected data (Bobak and Leon, 1999). Figure 7.3 shows data on the annual prevalence of low birthweight (<2500 g) and geometric mean concentration of sulphur dioxide plotted for the 85 administrative districts of the Czech Republic.

1. Looking at Figure 7.3, was there an association between sulphur dioxide concentration and prevalence of low birthweight for the shaded districts?
2. A logistic regression model was used to estimate associations, adjusting for socio-economic factors at the district level. An odds ratio for low birthweight of 1.10 (95% CI: 1.02–1.17) and an odds ratio for stillbirths of 0.98 (95% CI: 0.80–1.20) were estimated for each 50 µg/m² increase in sulphur dioxide pollution. Interpret these results in relation to whether there is an epidemiological association between the exposure and each outcome.

Limitations of ecological studies

Apart from the issue of ecological fallacy, ecological studies are also prone to bias and confounding. The choice of study sample is often defined by the availability and quality of routinely collected data. Data may be collected differently in different settings, and diagnostic criteria and technologies can change over time, leading to differential misclassification. For example, hospital records may vary according to institution, and using these to compare outcome frequencies for different hospital catchment areas will subject the analysis to inherent selection and information bias of each hospital's record-keeping systems. Geographical comparisons may suffer from migration of populations between groups

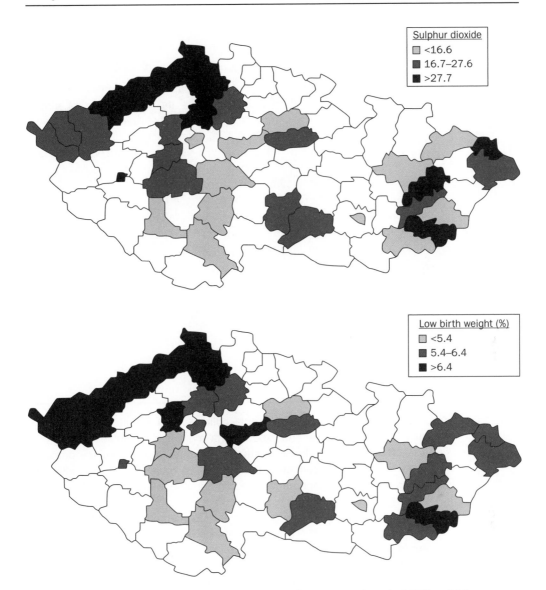

Figure 7.3 (a) Annual geometric mean sulphur dioxide concentrations in 1987 and (b) prevalence of low birthweight (<2500 g) in districts for which data were available

Note: No data available for unshaded areas.

Source: Bobak and Leon (1999).

over the period of the study, which may dilute any difference between groups. Finally, data are often collected for purposes other than epidemiological research and at a group level data on potential confounding factors are often missing.

✏️ **Activity 7.2**

Since 1995, paracetamol (acetaminophen) has been prescribed for use in neonates undergoing circumcision within the first 4 days of life. A study had the aim of exploring the relationship between early neonatal paracetamol exposure to autism and autism spectrum disorder (ASD), using circumcision as a proxy measure (Bauer and Kriebel, 2013). The population weighted average male autism/ASD prevalence and male circumcision rates were compared for nine countries after 1995. This showed an increase in autism/ASD prevalence of 0.20% for every 10% increase in circumcision prevalence ($r = 0.98$). A comparison of 12 countries before 1995 found an increase in autism/ASD of 0.04% for every 10% increase in circumcision prevalence ($r = 0.89$).

1. Interpret these results.
2. Given a growing body of experimental and clinical evidence linking paracetamol metabolism to autism and ASD, what would you conclude from these data?

Cross-sectional studies

An analytical cross-sectional study collects data simultaneously on the prevalence of outcome and exposure for a given study subject. Therefore, it is often difficult to know whether the exposure preceded the outcome and we cannot infer causality. For this reason, cross-sectional studies are generally used for generating research hypotheses and for health service planning and monitoring.

The appropriate measure of association is the *prevalence ratio*, however, if the outcome is rare (i.e. the prevalence is low), the prevalence ratio is approximately the same as the odds ratio (see pp. 42–4). This is useful, because it means that we can use logistic regression models to analyse cross-sectional studies, adjusting for several potential confounders, and report results as odds ratios.

Advantages of cross-sectional studies

This type of study measures prevalent cases and is best for measuring the frequency of chronic outcomes or markers of previous infection (e.g. antibodies). This means that it is generally rapid because there is no need to wait for sufficient incident cases to occur. However, cross-sectional studies may recruit participants over a longer period for less common outcomes. Because all data on an individual are collected simultaneously, it is logistically easier to include large numbers of individuals, who would ideally be sampled randomly to be representative of the population.

Cross-sectional studies allow for the collection of data on many variables, including several potential exposures. These studies are especially appropriate if the exposure status cannot change over time (e.g. genetic factors). They are also ideal for collecting data on potential confounders for use at the analytical stage.

Activity 7.3

Neisseria meningitidis infection is usually asymptomatically carried, with rare cases of meningitis and septicaemia. Twenty cross-sectional surveys were conducted in seven countries in the African meningitis belt. Table 7.2 shows selected results from the combined surveys, and from logistic regression analyses.

1. Calculate the prevalence of *N. meningitidis* carriage during the rainy and dry seasons.
2. Calculate an appropriate crude measure of association between *N. meningitidis* carriage and season of survey, comparing the dry with rainy season, and interpret the result.
3. Compare your result with that presented in Table 7.2, and explain the difference.
4. Interpret the adjusted odds ratios for recent meningitis vaccination in Table 7.2.

Table 7.2 Combined results of *N. meningitidis* carriage from 20 surveys, and odds ratios (OR) from multivariable logistic regression analyses with 95% confidence intervals (95% CI)

Factor	Subjects (Carriers)	Adjusted OR (95% CI)*
Season		
Rainy	32,978 (1039)	1.0
Dry	15,512 (648)	1.54 (1.37–1.75)
Recent meningitis vaccination		
No	33,598 (1230)	1.0
Yes, <1 year ago	9132 (227)	0.67 (0.57–0.78)
Yes, 1–3 years ago	4589 (171)	1.01 (0.85–1.21)

*Adjusted for potential confounders, such as age, sex, country.

Source: Selected data from Menafricar (2015).

Limitations of cross-sectional studies

It is often not possible to know whether the exposure preceded the outcome, and some outcomes have long latent periods. For example, the time between exposure to HIV and onset of AIDS can be more than 10 years. Therefore, a cross-sectional study would not have been appropriate to investigate an association between HIV infection and AIDS prevalence in the early days of the AIDS epidemic.

Measurement of current exposure may not be appropriate if the exposure may change over time, particularly in response to the outcome – known as **reverse causality**. For example, people with colon cancer may adapt the foods they eat to reduce discomfort, so current diet would not be a reasonable proxy for previous diet as a risk factor.

Recording exposure through self-reported history may suffer from recall bias. Therefore, measures of past exposure from routine data (e.g. health records if accessible) or more memorable exposures (e.g. occupation, previous smoking habits) are more appropriate.

Activity 7.4

A survey of adolescents aged 12–16 years was undertaken in Goa, India, using a development and well-being assessment to diagnose the presence of mental disorders. Structured interviews were conducted to assess risk factors, including family relations in the previous 12 months. Eligible individuals were identified through health centre family registers and a door-to-door survey. Of 2648 eligible adolescents, 358 were absent from home on three visits by the researcher, 85 had migrated, 187 did not consent to participate, and 6 did not complete the assessment. Of the 2048 analysed, 37 were diagnosed as having a mental disorder. Selected results of multiple logistic regression analyses are shown in Table 7.3.

Table 7.3 Factors associated with the presence of a mental disorder in adolescents

Risk factor	Odds ratio (95% CI)	P-value
Physical/verbal abuse from parents		0.02
Never/rarely	1.00	
Occasionally	1.50 (0.60–3.70)	
Often	2.90 (1.30–6.80)	

Table 7.3 *(continued)*

Risk factor	Odds ratio (95% CI)	P-value
Perceived family support		0.01
Rarely	1.00	
Sometimes	0.18 (0.10–0.70)	
Often	0.15 (0.04–0.50)	
Always	0.16 (0.10–0.50)	

Source: Selected data from Pillai et al. (2008).

1. What are the two hypotheses being tested in Table 7.3? [*Note*: The 'reference' or unexposed group is that with an odds ratio of 1.00.]
2. Interpret the results in Table 7.3, referring to any trends in odds ratios, 95% confidence intervals, and *P*-values.
3. What potential sources of bias can you identify from the information given, and how might these affect interpretation of the results?

Cohort studies

Epidemiologists use the term cohort to describe a group of individuals who share a common characteristic and are followed over time to measure the incidence of an outcome. A cohort may be a group of workers from a factory, a group of children who were born in the same year, or a group of individuals at risk of an outcome. Cohort studies measure the exposure of interest, and form a type of natural experiment observing the progression from exposure to outcome over time. This is usually considered the best analytical design to infer causality, as the definition of exposure prior to outcome meets the temporality criterion (see Chapter 4) and may reduce problems of information and selection bias. Cohort studies are most often used when the outcome of interest is common, as a rare outcome would require too large a sample size.

Cohort studies are also known as 'incidence studies', 'longitudinal studies' or 'follow-up studies', and categorize the cohort based on exposure status. Data on exposures that are not going to change during the study, such as date of birth, birthweight, adult height, blood type, and genetic factors are collected when participants enter the study through a descriptive cross-sectional survey. Exposures subject to change (e.g. blood pressure, physical activity, smoking, disease status) are collected by re-assessing individuals in the cohort at predefined time points during the study, or sometimes from medical records as and when they occur. If data on the exposure are detailed, there may be an opportunity to study dose–response relationships between exposure and outcome. Detailed information on confounding factors can also be collected, allowing investigators to control for them in the analysis. Data on outcomes may be collected through periodic health examinations, health outcome questionnaires administered to members of the cohort, consulting medical records, or using other forms of routine data.

It can be helpful to present the flow of numbers of study participants when describing a cohort study (see Figure 7.4). Most cohort studies are **prospective cohorts**, following participants over time until they either acquire the outcome of interest or the time limit for the study is reached. Study participants must usually be free of the outcome of interest at the start of the study. For example, if the outcome is having cancer, it is important to ensure that no participants have a cancer diagnosis at the start of the study.

Retrospective cohort studies use pre-existing data on exposures and outcomes (e.g. medical or occupational records, death notifications) and do not need to follow individuals over time, as the outcome information is already available. These are usually quicker and cheaper to conduct than prospective studies, particularly for diseases or events that may take decades to develop (e.g. cancer). However, routine data may be poorly collected (e.g. inaccurate, missing data), may not provide necessary information on other important risk factors or confounders, and may be liable to changes in definitions and coding systems over time. A cohort study may combine both retrospective and prospective data. For example, a study may identify a cohort of children aged 2 years and follow them for a year to measure the incidence of vaccine preventable diseases, while using vaccination records that pre-date the start of the study to provide information on prior exposures.

In an analytical cohort study, the appropriate measure of epidemiological association is the risk ratio or incidence rate ratio, depending on the

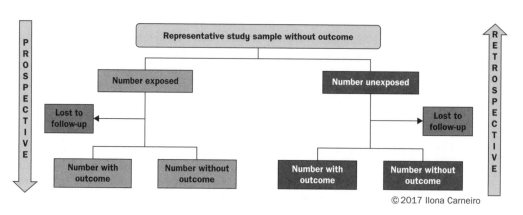

© 2017 Ilona Carneiro

Figure 7.4 Template flowchart for a cohort study

Note: Shows numbers recruited, categorized as exposed or unexposed, lost to follow-up in each category, and those with and without the outcome in each exposure category at the end of the study.

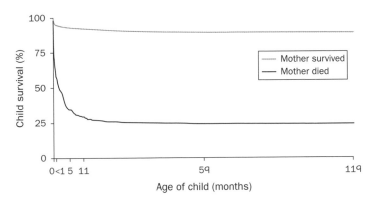

Figure 7.5 Survival curve from birth according to survival status of mother
Source: Ronsmans et al. (2010).

frequency measure used, and regression models allow us to adjust for the effect of potential confounders. If outcome frequencies are being compared between two cohorts that do not have the same population structure (e.g. the study cohort and the general population), it may be necessary to standardize the data first (see Chapter 6).

As some exposures may vary over time, it is important that any changes in exposure status are recorded and updated. A more complex statistical technique called 'time-series analysis' can be used to take account of changes in exposure, timing of outcome, and more detailed changes in person-time at risk (e.g. temporary movement out of the study area). Results of such analyses may be presented graphically as a survival curve or a failure curve, sometimes called Kaplan-Meier graphs. Such graphs can be used for any outcome, where failure represents acquisition of the outcome (e.g. incidence of cancer) and survival represents the lack of outcome (e.g. those *not* rejecting an organ after a transplant operation). Figure 7.5 shows a child survival curve from a cohort study in rural Bangladesh, comparing those whose mother had died before the child's tenth birthday to those whose mother had not. The distance between the two lines provides a graphical representation of the relative effect of maternal mortality and enables us to see how the effect changed over time (in this case, by the child's age in first year of life).

Advantages of cohort studies

Cohort studies enable us to study a wide range of outcomes that may be associated with a single exposure of interest. Even an outcome that was not anticipated at the start of the study may be included in data collection subsequently. This is especially useful when dealing with the introduction of new exposures whose health risks are undefined (e.g. mobile phone use, wireless technologies), and information on exposures can also be updated during the study.

Selection of the study population usually depends on whether the exposure of interest is common or rare. If the exposure is common, selection of the cohort depends on the group being disease-free at the start of the study. We can select a random sample from the general population before classifying everyone as exposed or unexposed. Alternatively, the study population could be selected from an occupation group (e.g. nurses, mine workers) or by place of work (e.g. factory). This is known as an 'occupational cohort' and has the advantage of higher participation and a higher level of follow-up than general population cohorts. For the purposes of measuring the association, it does not matter that the workforce cohort is not representative of the general population, just that the exposed and unexposed groups within the cohort are comparable to one another.

If the exposure is rare, the study sample can be selected according to exposure to ensure that enough exposed people are included to make the study viable. For example, if the exposure of interest is contact with industrial chemicals, then workers at a factory known to handle chemicals as part of their job can be chosen as the exposure group. The comparison group would then be selected from workers at the same factory who did not work with those chemicals. This is known as an 'internal comparison group', and is useful when looking to provide recommendations for appropriate occupational regulations. For example, for an occupational cohort of asbestos removal workers, we can investigate the risks of lung cancer associated with the type of respirator used and number of exposure hours, rather than just the occupation per se.

If we were looking at a risk factor to which the whole workforce had some degree of exposure, we would need to select a comparison group from another workforce as an 'external comparison group'. The use of another workforce aims to avoid the 'healthy worker effect', a form of selection bias that tends to underestimate **excess risk** associated with an occupation by comparing it with the general population, which includes people who are too sick to work.

✐ Activity 7.5

A cohort of employees aged 35–50 years was established in 1989 at a French company where individuals typically remain until retiring at age 55–60 years, after which they receive a company pension (Westerlund et al., 2010). Participants completed annual questionnaires about chronic diseases, perceived fatigue, and depressive symptoms for up to 7 years before and after retirement. Data were analysed on 14,104 out of 18,884 individuals retiring between 1990 and 2006, excluding those who retired on health grounds or with too many missing questionnaires. The cumulative prevalence of chronic diseases increased with age, with no break in the trend around the time of retirement. However, while perceived fatigue and depressive symptoms increased gradually with age, they showed a drastic change around the time of retirement. Logistic regression comparing one year after (exposed) with one year before retirement (unexposed) gave the following results: mental fatigue (odds ratio (OR) = 0.19; 95% CI: 0.18–0.21), physical fatigue (OR = 0.27; 95% CI: 0.26–0.30), and depressive symptoms (OR = 0.60; 95% CI: 0.53–0.67).

1. Explain the benefits and limitations of this study for measuring the effect of retirement on these outcomes.
2. Interpret the results presented.
3. The UK government is planning to raise the retirement age from 65 to 66 by 2020 and to 67 by 2028. What implications might this study have for UK policy?

Limitations of cohort studies

The length of follow-up needed for a sufficient proportion of the participants to have acquired an outcome may be many years (even decades for more rare outcomes). This can make cohort studies expensive and time-consuming to conduct if an active **follow-up** is used (e.g. regular health evaluations, quality-of-life questionnaires). The use of passive follow-up through routine data (e.g. death or cancer notifications) is cheaper and easier when record-keeping systems are good (e.g. occupational cohorts).

Large numbers of participants may be required, and the required sample size is related to the amount of time that participants are followed up. For example, if the sample size required for a study is calculated as 1000 person-years at risk, the study could follow up 1000 people for one year, or 500 people for 2 years, or 250 people for 4 years. However, a longer follow-up time implies a greater likelihood of loss of contact with participants. This 'loss to follow-up' needs to be accounted for by increasing the initial sample size to cover expected losses. Therefore, if we expect to lose contact with 10% of participants over the course of a 2-year study, the number of participants recruited at the start of the study should be 10% higher than the sample size required.

High rates of loss to follow-up or differences in the loss to follow-up between exposure groups can lead to selection bias. For example, if long-term follow-up is conducted by a self-completed questionnaire, participants may be less likely to respond due to death, disability, moving into a nursing home, etc.

The observational nature of the cohort design may sometimes raise ethical conflicts when dealing with severe and potentially fatal outcomes, as any interference by the investigator would have an impact on the outcomes being measured. Such issues need to be considered as part of the study design.

✎ Activity 7.6

The British Doctors' Study is an important prospective cohort study, which has followed participants for 60 years to investigate the relationship between tobacco smoking and cause-specific mortality among British doctors. In 1951, a questionnaire on smoking habits was sent to 49,913 male and 10,323 female doctors registered with the British General Medical Council; 34,440 male doctors and 6194 female doctors gave sufficient information to classify their smoking status (Doll and Peto, 1976; Doll et al., 1980). The vital status of these doctors was followed up from the records of the Registrar General's Office, the British Medical Council, and the British Medical Association. The causes of death for 10,072 male and 1094 female doctors who had died during the first 20 and 22 years of follow-up respectively were ascertained from death certificates. The rate of death from lung cancer among smokers was compared with that among non-smokers.

1. Discuss the potential sources of bias in this study.
2. Identify what information on smoking you would collect to classify tobacco smoking exposure status.
3. Age-adjusted lung cancer death rates per 100,000 persons per year among smokers and non-smokers in male and female doctors are given in Table 7.4. Calculate appropriate epidemiological measures of association between smoking and lung cancer for each level of exposure.
4. Discuss the results from part (3), especially the differences between males and females.

Table 7.4 Lung cancer death rates per 100,000 person-years by gender and smoking status

Gender	Non-smokers	Smoking 1–14 cigarettes/day	Smoking 15–24 cigarettes/day	Smoking 25+ cigarettes/day
Male	10	78	127	251
Female	7	9	45	208

Source: Selected data from: Doll and Peto (1976) and Doll et al. (1980).

Case-control studies

While recruitment of participants may be prospective, case-control studies are inherently retrospective because they define study groups by outcome and compare previous exposure to risk factors. Individuals are selected based on whether they do (**case**) or do not (**control**) have the outcome, and it is not possible to estimate the frequency (i.e. prevalence, risk, **odds** or incidence rate) of the outcome in the target population from case-control data.

This study design is especially useful for studying rare outcomes, as cases are preferentially identified so the sample size can be smaller and there is no need for lengthy follow-up. This results in a faster and cheaper design than cohort studies, making it a common choice for researchers. However, case-control studies are susceptible to selection and information bias, and a poor study design may lead to incorrect conclusions.

One way to reduce confounding of the association between exposure and outcome is to identify controls with the same characteristics as the cases, known as **matching**. 'Individual matching' identifies between one and four controls for each case, of the same age or gender. Other potential confounders, such as place of residence or ethnicity may be used, depending on the study aims. An alternative is 'frequency matching', where the controls are selected to be like the cases regarding the matched variable. To frequency-match by gender, for example, if our cases were 60% female, we select a control group that was also 60% female. However, matching can be more complicated and costly, and is not necessary if sufficient data on potential confounders are collected to enable adjustment during analysis.

A special type of design is the **nested case-control study**, where the case-control study is 'nested within' an existing cohort. In this design, cases are members of the cohort that have developed the outcome, and controls are members of the cohort without the outcome. This reduces selection biases that are inherent in simple case-control studies. It also reduces confounding by matching on factors common to all cohort members; for example, in an occupational cohort study, cases and controls will automatically be matched on employment status. This study design also means that new hypotheses can be tested more easily, since data on exposures are likely to have been collected as part of the cohort study, which will save time and money. As data on exposures may have been collected prior to the outcome, there is less chance of recall and observer bias, and it is easier to establish the temporal condition for causality. However, depending on what the cohort was designed for, there may be limited data on relevant exposures or other study design issues.

The outcome measure for a case-control study is the odds ratio (OR) of exposure (see Chapter 3), which is the odds of exposure in cases divided by the odds of exposure in controls. This has the same numerical value as the odds ratio of outcome, although the interpretation is different. For example, in a case-control study measuring the association between stress and traffic accidents, an odds ratio of 1.82 indicates that cases (individuals in a traffic accident) have 82% greater odds of exposure to stress than controls. It does not mean that those who reported stress had an 82% greater risk of being in an accident, although odds ratios of exposure and outcome are often incorrectly used interchangeably.

If the study is matched, then a more complicated analysis needs to be performed to account for matching. In this type of analysis, only the matched groups that are discordant (i.e. where either the case is exposed and the control unexposed, or the case is unexposed and the control exposed) are compared to give the matched odds ratio of exposure. This is because pairs where both case and control are exposed, or both case and control are unexposed, provide no information on differences in exposure. This can be done using 'conditional logistic regression', allowing adjustment for potential confounders.

Activity 7.7

Two prospective cohorts of nurses were followed up over a 10-year period and blood samples were collected at specified time points. Of 62,439 women participants, 144 with definite or probable multiple sclerosis (MS) and 288 healthy age-matched women were identified for inclusion in a new study (Ascherio et al., 2001). Blood samples were tested for antibodies to Epstein Barr virus (EBV) and cytomegalovirus (CMV). The researchers reported a relative risk of 1.7 (95% CI: 1.3–2.3) for antibodies to EBV and 0.9 (95% CI: 0.7–1.1) for antibodies to CMV, in samples collected after disease onset.

1. What type of epidemiological study is this? Be as specific as you can.
2. Interpret these results.

Advantages of case-control studies

As participants are selected according to their outcome status, it is possible to recruit the minimum number of cases and controls required before the study begins. The case-control design is useful when a rapid result is required, as with outbreak investigations or the appearance of a new syndrome (e.g. AIDS).

Case-control studies are more efficient than cohort studies when there is a long period of time between the exposure and outcome (latency period), as for chronic diseases such as cancer. As exposure is classified after the outcome, it is also possible to investigate the association of an outcome with multiple exposures.

Case-control studies are especially useful in genetic epidemiology (Khoury and Beaty, 1994), where the interaction between genetic and environmental factors is investigated, because genes do not change with time. The sequencing of the human genome has led to the search for disease susceptibility genes, and the case-control design enables investigation of several genetic markers (and potentially the whole genome) in the same study. In addition, genetic mutations are rare, requiring clinical and laboratory tests that would be prohibitively expensive in a cohort study. Familial aggregation studies may use the case-control design to identify clustering of an outcome within families, where the exposure will be family history of the outcome. Note that gender, ethnicity, and other forms of population structuring are likely to be confounders in studies of genetic traits and outcomes.

✎ Activity 7.8

In May 1997, a 3-year-old boy died of a respiratory illness labelled as 'avian' influenza A (H5N1). A case-control study was carried out in Hong Kong in January 1998 to identify risk factors for an outbreak of influenza A (H5N1) after 15 patients were hospitalized with the disease (Mounts et al., 1999). Two age- and gender-matched controls were identified for each case by randomly selecting a neighbouring apartment building to each case's residence and asking for volunteers.

1. Discuss the benefits and limitations of using a case-control design in this situation.
2. Interpret the investigators' main finding of an odds ratio of 4.50 (95% CI: 1.20–21.70) for exposure to live poultry in the market the week before illness, and consider the implications.

Limitations of case-control studies

Case-control studies are prone to many biases. The case definition must be very precise, and inclusion and exclusion criteria must be clearly stated before the study is conducted to ensure that case diagnosis is kept uniform throughout the study.

An important consideration is the source of cases; for example, if an outcome is particularly severe, cases may be found only in hospitals. If the outcome is rare or unusual, it is important to make sure that all locations of patients are identified, as patients may travel out of their local hospital catchment area to get specialist treatment at, for example, a referral hospital.

To reduce selection bias, it is essential that controls come from the same population as cases, but also that choice of controls is independent of the exposure of interest. If there is bias in who reaches hospital, then it may be appropriate to recruit controls from among other hospital patients, if their selection is not then biased in terms of the exposure of interest. For example, we may want to investigate risk factors for liver cirrhosis. If we suspect heavy alcohol use to be a major risk factor and select cases from hospital records, we may have problems if our hospital-based controls include a large proportion of people admitted to hospital for trauma. As people admitted for trauma are more likely to be heavy users of alcohol than the general population, this would bias the control group and reduce the ability to detect any increased exposure among cases. If all people with an outcome go to hospital, and there is no other distortion involved in the cases reaching hospital other than the outcome and the exposures under consideration, then controls can be selected from the general population.

If cases can be easily identified from the general population, then controls can be randomly selected from the same population with less likelihood of selection bias. Controls should meet all the criteria for cases (i.e. be as similar as possible), except for the outcome itself. For example, if the cases are men aged 40–65 years with lung cancer, the controls should be selected from men of that age group who do not have lung cancer.

It is necessary to consider whether both incident and prevalent cases should be included. Inclusion of prevalent cases may make it easier to generalize the study to the target population. However, prevalent cases may differ from incident cases in ways that may reduce the validity of the study. Inclusion of prevalent cases, especially for chronic outcomes, can create problems for determining exposure to certain risk factors that may change over time, leading to reverse causality.

Inclusion of prevalent cases may also lead to under-representation of more severe cases of a rapidly progressive outcome, who will die sooner after diagnosis and are less likely to be selected for the study. This in turn may affect the associations being investigated, as exposures associated with increased survival may be apparently associated with the outcome, even though they might be protective against the development of severe disease. If the outcome is fatal, it is important to ensure that patients who have died are included in studies using prevalent cases, to avoid selection bias.

Although matching can reduce confounding, it is important not to select too many characteristics on which to match, and not to select factors that might be very closely associated with exposure status. This can lead to **overmatching**, such that cases and controls do not differ sufficiently in relation to the main exposure of interest and we cannot measure the association. For example, in an early case-control study of AIDS, investigators compared cases with two age-matched HIV-negative homosexual male control groups (Moss et al., 1987). The first control was selected from the same neighbourhood as each case, while the second control was selected from those attending a clinic for sexually transmitted infections (STIs). The study found that cases were 52 times more likely to have >100 vs 0–5 sexual partners in the previous year compared with neighbourhood controls, but only 2.9 times more likely when compared with clinic controls. This is because STIs are associated with number of sexual partners, so clinic controls were biased towards having more partners and were overmatched on this exposure.

Reporting bias is more likely in case-control than other studies, as knowledge of being a case (or control) may affect what individuals remember, or how they report events or exposures. Cases may be more likely to remember events that occurred at around the time they were diagnosed with disease or underwent a traumatic event. For example, parents of children who develop autism may be more likely than other parents to remember the date of a vaccination, if it occurred in the days preceding a change in their child's behaviour. It is therefore important to use routinely collected data, or memory guides and prompts, when collecting data on exposure. Those collecting the exposure data (e.g. from interviews, medical records, biological samples) should ideally be unaware of the case or control status of the study participant, so avoiding observer bias.

✎ Activity 7.9

A case-control study aimed to measure the association between use of cannabis and the risk of psychotic disorders. In total, 410 patients aged 18–65 years with first-episode psychosis were recruited at health facilities in South London, with 24% refusal to participate among eligible patients. Also, 370 local population controls were identified through advertisements and the distribution of leaflets requesting volunteers, with no mention of drug use. All participants were administered a questionnaire to obtain socio-demographic data and information on the use of cannabis: 135 cases reported never having used cannabis compared with 138 controls.

1. Calculate an appropriate measure of association between lifetime history of cannabis use (ever vs never) and first-episode psychosis, and interpret your result.
2. Interpret the results presented in Table 7.5 on the effect of frequency of cannabis use on psychosis.
3. Use Table 7.5 to calculate the increased risk of first-episode psychosis with higher compared with lower potency cannabis use.

4. What other information might be relevant to include in the question-naire?
5. Does this study provide evidence of a causal association between cannabis use and psychosis?

Table 7.5 Cannabis use by outcome with adjusted odds ratios (OR) and 95% confidence intervals (95% CI) from logistic regression

Variable	Cases	Controls	Adjusted OR* (95% CI)
Frequency of consistent use			
Never used	135	138	1
<1 per week	68	128	0.58 (0.25–1.32)
At weekends	84	63	1.04 (0.41–1.62)
Every day	123	41	3.04 (1.91–7.76)
Most used type			
Never used	135	138	1
Hash-like (lower potency)	57	162	0.83 (0.52–1.77)
Skunk-like (higher potency)	218	70	2.91 (1.52–3.60)

* Adjusted for age, gender, ethnic origin, etc.

Source: Selected data from Di Forti et al. (2015).

Conclusion

In this chapter, we have reviewed the key features, advantages, and limitations of the main epidemiological analytical designs: ecological, cross-sectional, cohort, and case-control studies. Ecological studies are preferred when analysing population-level risk factors, or when comparing national or sub-national populations. Cross-sectional studies are usually cost-effective and useful for preliminary identifica-tion of epidemiological associations. Cohort studies are the most appropriate observational study design for investigating causality, but tend to be large and expensive. Case-control studies are espe-cially useful for studying rare outcomes, or those with long latency periods, but have a high likelihood of bias. The final choice of study design will often depend on the availability of data, together with logistics and funding.

Feedback on activities in Chapter 7

Feedback on Activity 7.1

1. The presentation of a map for each variable is descriptive rather than analytical, but we can see that both sulphur dioxide pollution and the prevalence of low birthweight were higher in the north-west and south-east districts, although the overlap is not perfect. This suggests that a relationship might exist, but requires an epidemiological analysis of the data.

2. The odds ratio for low birthweight is 1.10, indicating a 10% increase in the annual prevalence of low birthweight for every 50 $\mu g/m^2$ increase in population exposure to sulphur dioxide pollution. The 95% CI was 1.02–1.17, meaning we can be 95% confident that the true estimate of the odds ratio lies within this range. The 95% CI does not include 1.00, meaning that the P-value will be less than 0.05 (i.e. less than 5% probability that this association has been observed by chance through sampling variation, suggesting a true association). However, this does not mean that individual exposure to sulphur dioxide will increase the risk of low birthweight in a pregnant mother, as we cannot separate the population and individual-level effects. The odds ratio for stillbirths is 0.98 and the 95% CI includes 1.00, so there is no evidence that population exposure to sulphur dioxide pollution affects the risk of stillbirths.

Feedback on Activity 7.2

1. This is an ecological study, comparing the linear correlation (as indicated by the r-value) between national-level prevalence of circumcision and male autism/ASD. Both correlation coefficients are greater than zero, indicating a positive correlation, i.e. the prevalence of male autism/ASD increases with circumcision at a national level. In the data after 1995, when we assume that neonates being circumcised routinely received paracetamol, the increased prevalence of autism/ASD was much more strongly related with circumcision than for the data before 1995. This is consistent with a spatial and temporal association between neonatal paracetamol use and autism/ASD prevalence at a population level. However, this cannot tell us anything about this association at the individual level.

2. These data provide further evidence to support an association between paracetamol and autism and, together with the suggestion of biological plausibility from the experimental and clinical evidence, this indicates that a cohort or case-control study of this association should be undertaken.

Feedback on Activity 7.3

1. The prevalence is calculated as the number of carriers divided by the total number surveyed. This was $1039 \div 32,978 = 0.032$ or 3.2% in the rainy season, and $648 \div 15,512 = 0.042$ or 4.2% in the dry season.

2. These are cross-sectional surveys, so carriage is of prevalent infections, and the appropriate measure of association will be the prevalence ratio. You may have calculated it from part (1) as $0.042 \div 0.032 = 1.31$ or from the original data as $(648 \div 15,512)/(1039 \div 32,978) = 1.326$ (without the rounding error). This indicates a 33% higher prevalence of *N. meningitidis* in the dry season compared with the rainy season.

3. The result presented in Table 7.2 is an odds ratio from a multivariable logistic regression. As the prevalence of meningitis carriage is low, the odds ratio is likely to approximate the prevalence ratio, so this would not explain the difference seen. The higher result of 1.54 presented in Table 7.2 has been adjusted for several confounders, suggesting that the original association between *N. meningitidis* carriage and season was confounded by other factors such as age, sex, country, etc. After adjusting for potential confounders, there was a 54% higher odds of carriage of *N. meningitidis* in the dry compared with rainy seasons.

4. After adjusting for potential confounders, there was a significantly lower odds of *N. meningitidis* carriage in those who had been vaccinated within the past year compared with those who had not been vaccinated recently (odds ratio = 0.67), which is significant at the $P < 0.05$ level as the 95% CI does not include 1.00. This suggests a **vaccine efficacy** of 33% ($1 - 0.67 = 0.33$) for vaccination in the previous year. There is no evidence of protection from less recent vaccination, as the odds ratio for *N. meningitidis* carriage in those who had been vaccinated 1–3 years previously was 1.01 compared with those who had not been vaccinated recently, and the 95% CI included 1.00.

Feedback on Activity 7.4

1. Hypothesis 1: 'The prevalence of mental disorder in adolescents in this population increases with more frequent physical or verbal abuse from parents', OR 'Prevalence of mental disorder is greater among adolescents exposed to occasional or frequent physical/verbal abuse from parents than those exposed to no or rare physical/verbal abuse from parents.'

Hypothesis 2: 'The prevalence of mental disorder in adolescents in this population *decreases* with more frequent family support', OR 'Prevalence is *lower* in adolescents who receive support from their family (sometimes/often/always) than in those rarely supported by their family.'

2. In Table 7.3, the odds ratio of mental disorders appears to increase with increasing frequency of physical/verbal abuse from parents. The overall *P*-value of 0.02 indicates that there is less than a 2% chance that this association would be observed if it did not truly exist. The 95% CI for 'occasional' abuse from parents is 0.6–3.7, which includes the value 1.00, therefore individuals in this category are not at a significantly increased risk of mental disorder than those in the 'never/rarely' category. However, the 95% CI for the 'often' category is 1.3–6.8, which does not include 1.00, indicating that adolescents 'often' exposed to abuse from parents have almost three times (odds ratio = 2.90) greater odds of mental disorder than those 'never/rarely' exposed to abuse from parents.

   The odds ratio of mental disorders is much lower in adolescents who reported family support 'sometimes', 'often' or 'always', compared with those who reported family support 'rarely'. The overall *P*-value of 0.01 means there is less than a 1% chance that this association would be observed if it did not truly exist. However, there does not appear to be much of a trend since all categories had similar odds ratios (0.18, 0.15, 0.16), and their 95% CIs overlapped with each other. This suggests that the measure of level of family support did not discriminate well between the different categories. All three categories of adolescents who reported some family support had 95% CIs that did not include 1.00, indicating that they were all significantly different from those who reported 'rarely' receiving family support. In summary, adolescents reporting some family support had between 82% and 85% lower odds of suffering from a mental disorder.

3. There is likely to be *selection bias*. The 358 absent adolescents, 187 who refused to consent, and 6 who did not complete assessment, may have been different from the individuals analysed in relation to outcome or exposures. As this sums to 20% of those eligible, such potential bias in the estimate of effect makes it difficult to generalize the results to the target population.

   There is likely to be *information bias*, as exposures were all self-reported. The investigators developed structured interviews that had previously been tested elsewhere, and interviewed a sibling for 36% of participants. Given the high levels of stigma associated with the topic, there may have been under-reporting of abuse by parents, which would be differential misclassification and could underestimate the association. There may also be 'reverse causality', if individuals with mental disorders have different perceptions of their interactions and are, for example, more prone to perceiving abuse by parents or lack of family support. This could lead to over-reporting of abuse, which would also be differential misclassification but lead to overestimating the association.

Feedback on Activity 7.5

1. An occupational cohort is most appropriate for looking at the effect of retirement, as this can happen only to those in work. Through the company pension plan, it would be easier to maintain contact with the cohort and reduce loss to follow-up after retirement. A cohort design reduces the effects of bias, as measurements are taken before the exposure (retirement) occurs. However, many people will know that they are going to retire, probably at least one year in advance, and this is likely to affect their responses about perceived outcomes, so there is likely to be some responder bias in this period. There may also have been some selection bias, as only 14,104/18,884 = 0.747 or 75% of questionnaires were included in the analysis. Those who did not complete sufficient questionnaires or who retired on health grounds are likely to be very different from those included in the analysis.

2. The results suggest that people were 81% less likely to suffer from mental fatigue and 73% less likely to suffer from physical fatigue in the year after retirement, compared with the year before retirement. They were also 40% less likely to suffer from depressive symptoms one year after retirement compared with one year before. All these results were highly statistically significant at $P < 0.05$ because the 95% CIs were narrow and did not include 1.00.

3. These results might suggest that a delay in retirement age could lead to an increase in physical and mental fatigue and depressive symptoms, resulting in reduced productivity among the older workforce. However, as these were all self-reported outcomes, they may suffer from reporting bias. This French study looked at people retiring around the ages of 55–60 years, and given the large increase in the burden of chronic disease with age, may not be generalizable to the much later UK retirement age.

Feedback on Activity 7.6

1. There are several potential sources of bias:

   - This is an occupational cohort, so estimates from the study may not be extrapolated directly to the general population, because of the *healthy worker effect*. Doctors are also likely to have had better access to good medical care than the general population.
   - There may be some *selection bias*. First, only 69% (34,400/49,913) of eligible male doctors and 60% (6194/10,323) of eligible female doctors gave sufficient information to be included in the cohort. Those who did not respond or gave incomplete information may have been different from those who did respond in a way that may also have affected their exposure or risk of outcome.

- It is unlikely that investigators could follow up all subjects for the full period, due to migration or loss of records (i.e. *loss to follow-up*). However, for this study, where the sample size is large and the routine reporting systems are robust, this is unlikely to have greatly affected the result.
- There may have been some *information bias*. First, if some doctors gave inaccurate information regarding their smoking habits, this could have resulted in misclassification of exposure to smoking. At the time of classification of exposure to smoking in 1951, the association with lung cancer was not commonly known. Some case-control studies had indicated an association, and some doctors may have been aware of this, but they would not have known their own future risk of lung cancer. Therefore, any such responder bias would probably result in *non-differential misclassification* and underestimate the strength of the association.
- There could have been *observer bias* if lung cancer was more frequently diagnosed or certified as the cause of death among smokers than among non-smokers. However, this is unlikely since doctors would probably have had access to good medical care and lung cancer can be diagnosed accurately using various radiographic and histological investigations. In addition, the cause of death was obtained from death certificates and not diagnosed by study investigators.

2. A simple categorization could be to classify individuals as current smokers, former smokers or lifelong non-smokers. However, the effect of smoking may vary by the age doctors started to smoke, age of stopping smoking for former smokers, type of smoke (i.e. cigarette, cigar, pipe), and a dose effect may be investigated by quantifying the amount smoked (i.e. number of cigarettes per day, inhalation of smoke, second-hand smoke). Information on as many of these variables as feasible should be collected, if it does not reduce compliance with the study.

3. As rates are given in Table 7.4, the appropriate measure of association is the incidence rate ratio (IRR) of lung cancer deaths among different categories of smokers for males and females (you may wish to refer to Chapter 3). It would be most appropriate to use the death rate in non-smokers as the reference 'unexposed' category. The IRR for lung cancer among males smoking 1–14 cigarettes per day compared with male non-smokers is calculated as: $78 \div 10 = 7.8$. Similarly, the IRR for lung cancer among females smoking 25+ cigarettes per day compared with female non-smokers is calculated as: $208 \div 7 = 29.7$. You should have calculated the remaining IRRs from Table 7.4 as shown in Table 7.6. Note, the IRR for the reference category is always 1.00.

Table 7.6 Results from question (3): incidence rate ratios for lung cancer death by gender and smoking status

Gender	Non-smokers	Smoking 1–14 cigarettes/day	Smoking 15–24 cigarettes/day	Smoking 25+ cigarettes/day
Male	1.00	7.8	12.7	25.1
Female	1.00	1.3	6.4	29.7

4. The IRR for lung cancer death increased with the quantity smoked among both male and female doctors. This dose–response effect lends support to a causal association between smoking and lung cancer.

   The IRR in men smoking 1–14 and 15–24 cigarettes per day is much higher than in women. In those smoking 25 or more cigarettes per day, the IRR in men is marginally less than that in women. Does this mean that the effect of low levels of smoking is higher among men than among women? Without carrying out statistical tests, we cannot know whether these IRRs are significantly different, but the study had a large sample size and the magnitude of difference is high, so it is unlikely to be due to chance. However, the number of cigarettes smoked is unlikely to be a sufficiently good estimate of overall exposure to tobacco, which will be affected by other factors as well, such as the age of starting smoking (which was later among women than men in this cohort) and inhalation (more men than women in this cohort reported inhaling). These other factors may modify the effect of number of cigarettes smoked on lung cancer death.

Feedback on Activity 7.7

1. This is a nested matched case-control study, with cases of MS and healthy age-matched controls identified from within two prospective occupational cohorts of female nurses.
2. As this is a case-control study, the appropriate measure of association is an odds ratio of exposure. These results indicate that women with MS were 1.7 times or 70% more likely to have antibodies to EBV than controls, and this was statistically significant at $P < 0.05$, as the 95% CI did not include 1. This suggests an association between MS and EBV infection, but as it was assessed after disease onset, we do not know which came first, and there could be some reverse causality. [*Note:* The authors showed that this association was even more pronounced from a subset of blood samples that were available prior to disease onset.]

   Women with MS were 10% less likely to have antibodies to CMV than controls, but the 95% CI included 1.00, indicating a non-significant result with greater than 5% probability that this difference was observed by chance.

Feedback on Activity 7.8

1. The case-control design is ideal for an outbreak, as rapid results are needed. There are unlikely to be many prevalent cases, so a cross-sectional study would be inappropriate. It is not possible to predict the frequency of the outcome, and when first identified the outcome is likely to be rare, making it impractical to implement a cohort study.

   However, there may be selection bias due to difficulties in identifying appropriate controls, especially if the risk factors have not yet been identified. The choice of neighbourhood controls could lead to overmatching if the risk factor is an environmental exposure, and several types of controls should be used in this situation to avoid this bias. There may be information bias, as the outcome status is already known. In this situation, where media coverage of the death had occurred and the source of the virus had been identified as birds, cases may have remembered their recent contact with live poultry differently to controls, thus biasing results.

2. As this is a case-control study, the measure of association is the odds ratio of exposure. This means that cases were four times more likely than controls to have had contact with live poultry in the week before their illness. As the 95% CI does not include 1, it suggests that this result is significant at the $P < 0.05$ level, although the CI is very wide and is close to 1. It is not an odds ratio of outcome, so does *not* tell us that those who had contact with live poultry were four times more likely to suffer from H5N1 disease.

   It is a useful indicator of an association between exposure to live poultry and the outcome, but has limitations as mentioned in part 1. Given the implications of identifying live poultry markets as the cause of the outbreak (e.g. slaughter of all poultry, closure of poultry markets), further supportive evidence would be needed (e.g. isolation of H5N1 virus from poultry in the markets) before inferring causality.

Feedback on Activity 7.9

1. As this is a case-control study, the appropriate measure of association is the odds ratio of exposure. The odds of ever using cannabis among cases would be (410 − 135) ÷ 135 =2.037; the odds of ever using cannabis among controls would be (370 − 138) ÷ 138 = 1.681. The odds ratio of exposure to lifetime cannabis use is 2.037 ÷ 1.681 = 1.21, or (275 ÷ 135)/(232 ÷ 138) = 1.21. This means that there are 21% increased odds of having ever used cannabis among cases of first-episode psychosis compared with population controls. [*Note*: This difference was not statistically significant.]

2. Assuming the risk of psychosis is relatively rare in the population, the odds ratio from a logistic regression will approximate the prevalence

ratio (these are prevalent cases of psychosis). The inclusion of 1.00 and the overlapping 95% CIs suggest that there is no significant difference in the prevalence of psychosis among those using cannabis at weekends or less than once per week, compared with those who have never used it. However, there was a three times greater prevalence of psychosis among those who reported using cannabis every day, compared with those who had never used it, and this was statistically significant at $P < 0.05$ as the 95% CI did not include 1.00.

3. The odds ratio of exposure to higher potency compared with lower potency cannabis use among cases compared with controls can be calculated as: $(218 \div 57)/(70 \div 162) = 8.85$. This suggests that among individuals who have used cannabis, those who suffer an episode of psychosis have more than eight times higher odds of having used higher potency cannabis than lower potency cannabis. However, this is a crude result and was not adjusted for any confounding effects.

4. Other information that might be relevant to include in the questionnaire are the age at which cannabis use started, the duration of cannabis use, and the amounts of cannabis used. Potential confounders would include use of tobacco, alcohol and other recreational drugs, socio-demographic factors (e.g. age, gender, ethnic origin, education, employment status), and information on family history of psychosis or other psychiatric illnesses.

5. Before supporting a causal association, we need to consider alternative explanations for the observed associations. The results for daily use of cannabis and for higher potency cannabis use are statistically significant at $P < 0.05$, suggesting that these associations are not due to chance. As this is a case-control study, there are several inherent biases. First, the exposure is determined after the outcome has occurred, so responder, reporting or recall bias may affect the cases' responses. Second, there was 24% refusal to participate by eligible cases, which could lead to selection bias if those refusing were different from those consenting. Third, controls were volunteers and not a random sample of the population, which may have led to selection bias, as they may not be representative of the general population. While several confounders were adjusted for in the analysis, there may still have been residual confounding or confounding by unknown factors. Evidence supporting causality would include the magnitude of effect (a 200% increased risk is large) and the suggestion of a dose-effect when frequency and potency are assessed. [*Note*: There is already supportive evidence from cohort studies (consistency) as well as experimental evidence (biological plausibility).] Overall, these data support a causal association between frequent use of cannabis and use of high potency cannabis with first-episode psychosis, but do not support an association between all cannabis use and psychosis.

Intervention studies $\boxed{8}$

Overview

The analytical study designs described in Chapter 7 are observational, and while a well-designed cohort study may support a causal association, the only way to determine causality is through intervention. Intervention studies are epidemiological experiments during which the investigators manipulate the exposure to see what effect it has on the outcome. In this chapter, you will learn that the **randomized controlled trial** (RCT) is the ideal design, as it can reduce error due to bias and confounding. However, given ethical and logistical constraints, other intervention study designs may be necessary when an RCT is not possible. Intervention studies may measure intervention efficacy under ideal trial conditions or effectiveness under routine conditions.

Learning objectives

When you have completed this chapter, you should be able to:

- describe the key features, strengths, and limitations of intervention studies
- discuss ethical issues related to the design and conduct of intervention studies
- define the main characteristics of randomized controlled trials
- recognize when non-randomized intervention studies may be appropriate
- differentiate between intention-to-treat and per-protocol analyses

What defines an intervention study?

An intervention study measures the association between an outcome and exposure to a specific intervention. An **intervention** may focus on prevention of exposure in those at risk of the outcome (e.g. insecticide-treated mosquito nets against malaria) or treatment to reduce mortality or severity in those who already have the outcome (e.g. interferon treatment of people with chronic hepatitis B to reduce progression to liver cancer). A preventive intervention may remove or reduce an assumed risk factor (e.g. health education to reduce recreational drug use), or it may introduce or increase an assumed protective factor (e.g. vaccination against meningitis).

Either cohort or cross-sectional methods may be used to measure the relative frequency of the outcome in those exposed and unexposed to the intervention under study. However, unlike the observational study designs described previously, intervention studies are experimental because the investigators define which study subjects are 'exposed' and which are 'unexposed'. For ethical reasons, experimental studies are restricted to evaluating exposures that reduce the frequency of a negative outcome.

Intervention studies may be classified according to several consecutive phases, derived from clinical research of medical interventions (e.g. drugs, vaccines, diagnostics, surgical procedures). Phase I trials apply the intervention to small numbers (2–100) of healthy volunteers to assess issues such as safety and tolerability. Phase II trials evaluate efficacy and safety in larger groups of about 100–300 people. Phase III trials aim to provide definitive evidence of efficacy in those at risk of the outcome and usually use a randomized controlled design. Phase IV trials monitor the routine use of an intervention to collect data on long-term efficacy and safety (e.g. pharmacovigilance). Most epidemiological studies will be Phase III, while routine surveillance will be akin to Phase IV (see Chapter 10).

Advantages of intervention studies

The intervention study design is ideal for inferring causality (see Chapter 4) because:

- The exposure is defined prior to development of the outcome, so the temporal sequence is established, satisfying the 'temporality' requirement for causality.
- If the intervention removes or reduces an exposure that results in a reduction in the outcome frequency, this 'reversibility' will support causality.
- Investigators can randomize study subjects to be exposed and unexposed to the intervention. If the number of subjects is large enough to reduce the effects of chance, this ensures that all known and *unknown* confounders are equally distributed between comparison groups (i.e. comparison groups are identical in all ways except for the intervention and there is no selection bias).
- Investigators may be able to conceal the **allocation** of the intervention from study subjects and from those measuring the outcome, reducing information bias.

Limitations of intervention studies

Intervention studies are not usually appropriate for the prevention of very rare outcomes, as they generally use cohort methods that would require a long follow-up time. However, it is possible to use multiple research centres or health facilities to accumulate sufficient cases more quickly – known as 'multi–centre' studies. If the outcome is chronic (e.g. hepatitis C infection), it may also be possible to measure the intervention effect using cross-sectional surveys with very large sample sizes.

Intervention studies are usually expensive to conduct. They may require a large study team and lengthy follow-up time to identify sufficient subjects with the outcome. There are usually additional costs of the intervention itself, as well as costs related to concealing the allocation (see below) and monitoring the safety of the intervention.

Selection bias may occur at enrolment, especially if there are risks of serious side-effects or a chance of not receiving active treatment for a medical condition. For example, an individual with asymptomatic chronic hepatitis B infection might be less willing to join a trial of treatment to suppress viral replication than an individual with abnormal liver function. Similarly, individuals with advanced cancer that have already tried existing treatments may be more willing to try a new experimental treatment. This selection may affect the estimate of efficacy if the intervention acts differently at different stages of disease, and it may not be appropriate to generalize the result to the wider target population (known as **external validity**).

Bias may also be introduced during the study if there is a difference in compliance or follow-up between the intervention arms. For example, partici-pants may be more likely to withdraw from a study if there are side-effects or if they feel the intervention is not working. There may also be differ-ences in compliance due to clinical deterioration or because a participant forgets to administer a placebo because they do not notice any benefit (e.g. a placebo mosquito repellent). Participants who are lost to follow-up or do not comply may be different from those who complete the study, and baseline data on important risk factors should be collected. The propor-tions of subjects lost to follow-up and others not included in the final analy-sis must be compared between the different intervention arms to help identify any selection bias that may reduce the **internal validity** of the trial.

Efficacy and effectiveness

There are two stages in evaluating an intervention that can be addressed using an intervention study design. **Efficacy** studies aim to measure the effect of the intervention under 'experimental' conditions, where maximum effort is put into intervention delivery. For example, participants in an infant vaccine trial may be reminded to attend for vaccination or even visited at home if they do not attend the vaccination clinic on time.

Once an intervention has been proven to be efficacious, it may be appro-priate to undertake an **effectiveness** study to measure the effect of the intervention under 'real-world' conditions. This is especially important for interventions that rely on fragile delivery systems (e.g. weak health infrastructure), or where long-term patient compliance is required. Measures of effectiveness of an intervention may be very different to estimates of efficacy, and provide a better indication of its likely impact when administered to the general population. However, there is a continuum of efficacy and effectiveness, as routine conditions will vary according to the setting.

In the infant vaccine example, effectiveness will depend on factors such as whether the vaccine is in stock and viable, whether caregivers bring infants for vaccination, infant age when attending, and the number of doses they receive. For a vaccine with 90% efficacy, if only 50% of those at risk of the outcome receive sufficient doses of viable vaccine at the correct time, the effectiveness could be closer to 45% ($0.9 \times 0.5 = 0.45$).

Ethical issues

If an intervention is already available to the public or in routine use, it may not be feasible to withdraw it from participants in the control group without providing an alternative, even if the safety or efficacy of the intervention is unknown or in doubt. For example, there is no evidence that prenatal ultrasound screening improves birth outcome and concerns have been raised about its potential long-term effects. However, routine ultrasound scans are an accepted part of obstetric care in developed countries and it would be difficult to recruit sufficient subjects to a randomized trial where routine ultrasound was withheld from the comparison group.

Ethical objections may be raised about withholding an intervention from the comparison group if the intervention has already been shown to be safe and effective in a previous study. However, it is not unusual for an initial study to show evidence of an effect, while subsequent studies in different settings give conflicting results. For example, observational studies showed a 50% reduction in coronary disease in post-menopausal women using hormone replacement therapy (HRT). HRT was subsequently prescribed for this purpose, but subsequent large RCTs found no evidence of effect, supporting the need to gather sufficient evidence before changing policy and practice. Ethical responsibility must be balanced against the need for sufficient and consistent epidemiological evidence, and a systematic review of existing evidence should be undertaken before developing any intervention study proposal.

It is therefore necessary to obtain 'ethical approval' (i.e. permission) from national and institutional ethical bodies prior to conducting any epidemiological investigation, but this is even more relevant for intervention studies, as investigators determine which intervention the participants receive. However, whether a study is judged to be ethical can vary greatly between countries and over time, as scientific knowledge and cultural norms evolve.

Intervention studies need to address questions of sufficient clinical or public health importance to justify their use. Ethical considerations will often drive the choice of specific study design (see below), as most designs involve withholding a potentially efficacious intervention from subjects allocated to the control arm during the study period. This can only happen if those in the control arm are not 'subject to additional risks of serious or irreversible harm as a result of not receiving the best proven intervention' (World Medical Association, 2013). The general population will eventually benefit if the study provides sufficient evidence of a protective intervention effect, and those who participated in the trial should be the first to benefit from such an intervention once the trial is over.

Activity 8.1

Hormone replacement therapy (HRT) is the reference treatment for hot flashes in menopausal women, reducing them by 80–90%. However, several studies have shown an association between HRT use and increased risk of breast cancer. An intervention trial aimed to compare the efficacy of a non-hormonal homeopathic treatment with a placebo for reducing hot flashes (Colau et al., 2012). Discuss the ethical issues raised by this trial.

Randomized controlled trials

The ideal intervention study design is a randomized controlled trial (RCT) defined by: (a) the existence of a contemporary comparison group of study subjects who do not receive the same intervention, known as the 'control' arm; and (b) the random allocation of study subjects to either intervention or control arms.

Figure 8.1 shows a standard RCT profile as advocated by the CONSORT Group (2010), identifying the progress of participants through the trial. Potential trial participants should be randomly selected to be representative of the population to which the intervention will ultimately be applied. Individuals are assessed for inclusion using clearly defined eligibility criteria, and informed consent must be obtained (see Chapter 5). Participants are then randomly allocated. To reduce bias, the intervention allocation should be concealed, so that neither participants nor investigators are aware of the allocation.

Choice of control type

Participants receiving the intervention of interest are compared with those not receiving the intervention of interest. This latter group is called the **control** arm. Depending on the intervention being evaluated, 'control'

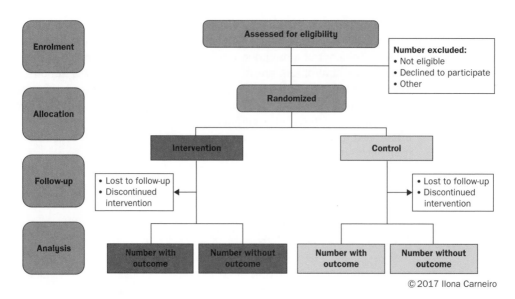

© 2017 Ilona Carneiro

Figure 8.1 Flow diagram of trial profile based on the CONSORT guidelines for reporting

subjects may receive (i) nothing, (ii) a **placebo** intervention, or (iii) an existing intervention. We usually want to know the effect of an intervention compared with current practice. If no intervention is currently in use, the control arm may receive no intervention, but should otherwise have identical access to treatment and preventive services as those in the intervention arm.

A placebo is a simulated intervention with no active properties, known as a negative control. Investigators may choose to use a placebo because the act of receiving an intervention may affect a subject's perceived or actual outcome. Individuals who think they are receiving a treatment may experience a reduction in symptoms. This positive outcome without any active intervention is known as the 'placebo effect'. A study subject may also experience more negative effects (i.e. increased symptoms or side-effects) after receiving a placebo, which is known as the 'nocebo effect'.

Brain imaging studies have shown that these responses have a neurobiological basis, but they are not yet fully understood. For some outcomes (e.g. Parkinson's disease, irritable bowel syndrome), self-healing processes were identified as playing a role after a placebo intervention was shown to have an effect. The use of a placebo enables us to adjust for the 'background' effects of participating in the trial, such as participant expectation, interaction with study investigators, and tests for monitoring and measuring the outcome. However, the 2013 World Medical Association 'Declaration of Helsinki' states that 'a new intervention must be tested against those of the best proven intervention' unless there are compelling methodological reasons to do otherwise, and cautions against unethical use of placebos.

The use of an existing intervention for comparison is known as an active or positive control. The control arm participants should receive the best current practice available to them, although this may not always be the best available worldwide. For example, studies in Country X find drug A to be a better treatment for tuberculosis than the existing drug B, and drug A is implemented as the new first-line therapy in Countries X and Y. However, no studies have yet been undertaken in Country Z where drug B is still the first-line therapy. Investigators may successfully argue for an RCT of drug A compared with drug B in Country Z, as control participants will be receiving the best *available* current practice. However, it would be difficult to carry out the same trial in Country Y, even if there were no prior local evidence, because drug A is already the best treatment currently available to study participants there.

Allocation

Participant allocation is usually randomized so that all study participants have an equal chance of being allocated to intervention or control arms, therefore avoiding 'allocation bias'. Intervention arms should have similar numbers of participants to reduce confounding. If the sample size is sufficiently large, randomization ensures that known and unknown confounding factors are equally distributed between study arms and will not interfere with the estimate of intervention effect. Random allocation can be undertaken using similar methods to those described for random sampling in Chapter 5, listed below in order of increasing complexity:

- *Simple randomization* could shuffle labelled cards or use a computer-generated random number list. However, this may result in different numbers of subjects in each study arm, and an imbalance in confounding factors if the sample size is small.
- *Systematic randomization* allocates participants to each group alternately (e.g. those attending clinic on specific days), but this may be subject to selection bias. For example, there may be systematic differences in the severity of patients presenting to a clinic on a Monday (after the weekend) and those presenting on a Tuesday.
- *Blocked randomization* restricts the allocation list to ensure equal numbers in all study arms, where the block size is a multiple of the number of treatment groups. For example, a trial comparing interventions A and B may use blocks of four to generate six possible randomization sequences with equal allocation probability: AABB, ABAB, BABA, ABBA, BAAB, BBAA. These can then be chosen at random to define the allocation sequence. However, this may be prone to allocation bias, as it may be possible for the investigator to predict and influence the allocation for the last few participants in each block.
- *Stratified randomization* divides participants into subgroups ('strata') based on key risk factors (e.g. age, gender), and equal numbers of

subjects from each stratum are then allocated to each study arm using simple or block randomization. This ensures that suspected confounders or effect modifiers of the association between intervention and outcome are equally distributed between comparison arms. For example, malaria incidence varies considerably between communities due to socio-economic and geographic differences. In an RCT of an infant malaria vaccine, infants should be stratified according to their village of residence prior to randomization. This allows the investigators to control for village-level differences in malaria risk and other factors.

- *Matched-pair randomization* is a form of stratified random allocation that matches individuals or communities into pairs with similar baseline risks of the outcome.

In small trials when several variables need to be balanced between study arms, stratified randomization is not sufficient to ensure comparability. Differences between study arms may still occur by chance, making it difficult to interpret results, even after adjusting for these differences in the analysis. In this situation, rather than randomly allocating subjects, we purposefully allocate them based on a pre-specified list of criteria. This is known as **minimization**, as the intention is to minimize differences between study arms. As each subject is enrolled, their allocation depends on the characteristics of those subjects already enrolled, and allocation is therefore somewhat predictable (for further details, see Altman and Bland, 2005).

For all the methods described above, there is a chance of conscious or unconscious selection bias if a study investigator undertakes the allocation, or if the patient knows which intervention they will receive and can then choose not to participate. For example, a clinician may tend to allocate more seriously affected patients to the intervention arm and less seriously affected patients to the control arm. Therefore, the allocation sequence should be concealed to reduce both allocation bias and selection bias. **Allocation concealment** may use sealed envelopes determining the allocation, which are opened only after an eligible subject has consented to enter the trial. For multi-centre trials, there may be a centralized system where subject details are entered on the trial computer, which then randomly allocates the subject to one of the treatment groups. Another method is for allocation to be done by the manufacturer of the intervention (e.g. drug, vaccine, mosquito net), with the intervention and control packaged identically with serial numbers whose coding is known only to the manufacturer.

Allocation concealment is not the same as **blinding** (see below). It is always possible to conceal the allocation sequence prior to allocation in RCTs, to prevent selection bias, even though it may not then be possible to conceal the allocation from participants or investigators during the trial.

Blinding

An 'open-label' trial is one where participants and investigators are aware of which intervention is allocated to which study subjects, and is common in Phase I and II studies. However, if participants know whether they are receiving a new intervention, existing intervention or placebo, it may affect their behaviour during the trial or responses to questions determining outcome. For example, a mother who knows her child was vaccinated against measles may be less likely to seek treatment for a fever than one whose child was not. If one of the study outcomes is clinic attendance with fever, this could result in information bias through differential case ascertainment between the study arms. This is of greater concern if the outcome may be subjective, such as reported improvement in symptoms of multiple sclerosis. Individuals receiving no intervention may also be unlikely to report any adverse effects (e.g. headaches), which may lead to an overestimate of adverse effects from the intervention.

Use of a placebo intervention can help to conceal the intervention allocation. While a placebo is easier to develop for drugs and vaccines, it is not impossible to develop placebos for non-chemical interventions, such as counselling or acupuncture, known as 'sham treatments'. For example, 'sham' surgery maintains the illusion of an operation by using real anaesthesia, surgical incision and pre- and postoperative care, but leaving out the actual intervention of interest. While this raises many ethical concerns, the increasing use of minimally invasive procedures (e.g. keyhole surgery) reduces negative effects for the participants while enabling the more rigorous testing of such interventions.

Observer bias can occur if the person assessing the outcome is aware of the allocation. For example, a microscopist reading blood slides to detect malaria parasites may be less thorough if they read the slides while sitting in a village with insecticide-treated curtains in every doorway than in one without curtains. For most outcomes, it is usually possible to 'blind' the observer – that is, to conceal the intervention allocation from the person diagnosing the outcome. It is important that intervention allocation is also blinded to those entering and analysing the data, to prevent any intentional or unintentional bias from being introduced at this stage.

If either participant or observer is blinded, the study is 'single-blind', whereas if both are blinded, the study is 'double-blind'. The gold standard epidemiological study is the double-blind, randomized placebo-controlled trial.

✎ Activity 8.2

A fictitious study was carried out on the maternity wards of 10 hospitals to test the effect of oral versus intramuscular vitamin K to reduce clinical bleeding in newborns. After obtaining informed parental consent, children born on odd-numbered days received doses of 2.0 mg oral vitamin K on days 1 and 3 after birth. Children born on even-numbered days constituted the control group and received 1.0 mg of intramuscular vitamin K the day after birth according to existing practice. All infants were followed up to assess spontaneous bleeding on days 1–7 after birth.

1. What type of study is this? Identify as many design characteristics as you can.
2. Discuss the potential limitations of this design and ways in which it might be improved.

More complex RCTs

Basic RCTs will randomize individuals to receive one of two treatments and assess which is better. However, we sometimes need more complex designs to answer a question more comprehensively. Community-level interventions are measured using a **cluster-randomized trial**, while a comparison of individual and combinations of interventions can be undertaken using a **factorial trial**. A **crossover trial** allows us to reduce the sample size and the effects of confounding for interventions that are not long-lasting. If we wish to compare an intervention that may be the same as, or no worse than, an existing intervention, we can use **equivalence** and **non-inferiority trials** respectively.

Cluster-randomized trials

In cluster-randomized RCTs, groups of individuals known as 'clusters' are randomly allocated to intervention and control arms, and all individuals within the same cluster receive the same intervention or control. This design may be used if the intervention acts at the cluster level; for example, an intervention that reduces air pollution would need to be introduced at the community level, since it would be impossible to introduce pollution controls at an individual level.

Cluster randomization may be appropriate when there is a risk of 'contamination' between the intervention and control groups, such that controls may be exposed to the intervention or vice versa – for example, in a trial of health education leaflets to promote healthy diet in school children, investigators would randomize at the school level. If they had randomized at the individual level, children within a school might show the leaflets to friends in the control group. Clusters must be sufficiently separated to prevent contamination – for example, an exclusion zone may be needed around treatment and control areas for a trial of indoor residual spraying with insecticide.

Individuals within a cluster will share several characteristics, which may lead to confounding. This can be overcome by using stratified allocation, together with block randomization to ensure a balance between intervention arms. As the individuals cannot be treated as independent observations, this leads to a reduction in statistical power and cluster-randomized trials require larger sample sizes. Special methods are required to estimate sample sizes for cluster-randomized trials and to analyse results (for more information, see Hayes and Moulton, 2009).

Factorial design

In a factorial trial, two or more interventions are compared individually and in combination against a control comparison group. This has the advantage of enabling us to assess interactions between interventions, and may save time and money by evaluating several intervention combinations simultaneously. For example, using a 2×2 factorial design results in a four-arm trial that compares individuals receiving both treatments with those receiving one or other of the two treatments and those receiving no treatment (the control group).

✐ Activity 8.3

A randomized factorial trial of falls prevention was undertaken among people aged 70 years and over, living in their own homes in urban Australia. Three interventions were compared: group-based exercise, home hazard management, and vision improvement. Table 8.1 presents the number having at least one fall over the 18-month study period.

1. Calculate appropriate measures of association to identify which individual intervention was most effective.
2. How much more effective was a combination of group-based exercise and improved vision than exercise alone?
3. What was the benefit of the factorial trial design, compared with a randomized trial of the complete package of three interventions?

Table 8.1 Results from a factorial trial of interventions on falls outcome

Intervention	Number of participants	Number having at least one fall
No intervention	137	87
Group-based exercise	135	76
Vision improvement	139	84

Table 8.1 *(continued)*

Intervention	Number of participants	Number having at least one fall
Home hazard management	136	78
Exercise + vision	136	66
Exercise + home hazard management	135	72
Vision + home hazard management	137	78
Exercise + vision + home hazard management	135	65

Source: Selected data from Day et al. (2002).

Crossover design

In a crossover design RCT, each trial subject (e.g. individual, village) acts as its own control by receiving either the intervention or control at different points in the study. A **washout period** (i.e. the time needed for the intervention to stop having an effect) is used to avoid contamination between the study periods, and may use no intervention or a third intervention if that is unethical. The order in which the subject receives the intervention or control (e.g. intervention then placebo or placebo then intervention) is determined by random allocation. This design enables us to control for confounders and effect modifiers, and a smaller sample size is needed because baseline characteristics are the same in the two arms. However, the crossover design is likely to be longer than a normal RCT, and there may be more dropouts or loss to follow-up. It is suitable only when the intervention does not have long-term effects, and may be especially appropriate for looking at short-term relief of symptoms or healthcare provider practice.

Non-inferiority and equivalence designs

While most intervention studies aim to identify whether an intervention is better than a placebo or existing treatment ('superiority trials'), sometimes the aim is to show that a new intervention is at least as good as ('non-inferior') or equal to ('equivalence') an existing intervention. For example, we may wish to test a cheaper drug against an existing expensive one, identify second-line treatments, alternatives with fewer adverse effects, or new methods of delivery. Finding that one intervention is not significantly better than another is not the same as proving that they are the same. There are many reasons for a non-significant difference, including sample size, bias, and confounding. These designs would use non-inferiority or equivalence null hypotheses to calculate the appropriate sample size required.

Non-randomized trials

Sometimes a non-randomized trial design is used to evaluate interventions by comparison with a historical, geographical or opportunistic control group, especially to measure effectiveness. While these studies are subject to bias and confounding, it is necessary to use these 'plausibility' designs to accumulate evidence on the impact of an intervention in situations where the intervention is very complex, evidence is required on a large scale, or ethical concerns prevent the use of an RCT (Victora et al., 2004). Standards complementing those of CONSORT have been developed to facilitate the Transparent Reporting of Evaluations with Nonrandomized Designs (TREND) (Centers for Disease Control and Prevention, 2017b) to facilitate evidence-based public health decisions.

Historical controls

If it is not possible to have a contemporary comparison arm for ethical or logistical reasons, an intervention study may compare outcome frequency before and after the intervention is introduced. This design is most commonly used in evaluations of health services, health promotion campaigns, and public health legislation (e.g. banning smoking in public places). However, the use of such 'historical' controls makes it difficult to distinguish the effect of the intervention from other changes that may have affected the outcome over the study period. If this design is used, it is necessary to carefully monitor other changes that may occur in the study population (e.g. migrations, introduction of other interventions, changes in climate variables), other outcomes that should not have been affected by the intervention, and the outcome of interest in the general population to which the intervention has not been applied.

Geographical controls

The use of communities or individuals as contemporary controls from outside the trial area may enable us to adjust for the effects of temporal changes during the evaluation. However, there are likely to be inherent differences between control and intervention communities that need to be considered when interpreting results.

A variant of this is the 'stepped-wedge' design, which is increasingly being used in the evaluation of service delivery interventions. It involves the phased introduction of an intervention to a population over time, usually in line with logistical constraints (e.g. time required for training of health staff or community health education). In the first such trial, hepatitis B vaccine was progressively introduced into The Gambia by adding a new immunization team responsible for a different part of the country every 3 months (The Gambia Hepatitis Study Group, 1987).

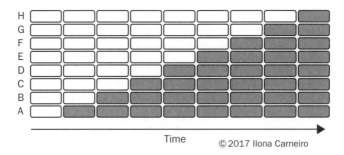

Time © 2017 Ilona Carneiro

Figure 8.2 Schematic of stepped-wedge intervention trial design applied progressively

Note: Shaded blocks represent clusters (A–H) receiving the intervention. Unshaded blocks represent clusters that have not yet received the intervention (controls).

Source: Based on Brown and Lilford (2006).

The intervention is usually applied at the cluster level, and allows for a crossover of each cluster from control to intervention, randomly allocating the order in which clusters introduce the intervention. Clusters that have not yet received the intervention act as the control arm of the study. Over the course of the trial, the total numbers of intervention and control clusters are equal, but the distribution varies with time (Figure 8. 2), and temporal trends in other risk factors may confound the findings. This can be reduced by having large numbers of clusters and small interval periods for introduction of the intervention to each additional cluster.

Opportunistic controls

This involves the use of individuals or communities that should have received the intervention but did not because the programme was unable to reach them. If the controls have varying degrees of exposure to the intervention, it may be possible to measure a dose–response effect. However, once more, there are likely to be many confounding factors that will need to be accounted for.

✏ **Activity 8.4**

Seasonal malaria chemoprevention (SMC) involving monthly administration of antimalarial drugs to children under 5 years during the malaria transmission season had high efficacy in clinical trials in areas with seasonal malaria transmission. SMC was introduced at primary care health posts in Senegal over a 3-year period, in a process requiring training and community education. A stepped-wedge cluster-randomized trial was undertaken to assess the effectiveness of SMC on the incidence of malaria in children identified at the health posts (Cisse et al., 2016).

1. Why do you think the authors chose this design rather than an individually randomized placebo-controlled design?
2. From the information given, what factors would need to be recorded and adjusted for in the analysis?

Analysis

It is good practice for a statistician independent of the study team to hold the concealment codes to the intervention allocation. Codes should not be revealed to study investigators until after data have been entered and cleaned. In large clinical trials, the data are 'frozen' (i.e. a copy of the data prior to 'breaking-the-code' is sent to an independent statistician for safekeeping) to ensure that data are not changed after the allocation is revealed.

A detailed analytical plan should be developed prior to breaking the allocation codes. This will state the primary outcome of interest, any secondary outcomes of interest, the methods of analysis to be used (e.g. logistic regression models), and any variables to be adjusted for in the analysis. This prevents investigators from searching through the data and only presenting positive results.

Interim analysis

In intervention studies with a long follow-up period, where there may be a possibility of severe adverse events, it is usual to have an independent trial safety monitoring board. This board is responsible for periodically reviewing all reports of severe adverse events. If there is a concern about greater than expected numbers of adverse events in one study arm, the board will analyse the data and, if necessary, the trial will be stopped. It is also common for the monitoring board to undertake an independent **interim analysis** of the data halfway through a long study. If there is sufficient epidemiological evidence that the intervention is working, or that the trial will have insufficient power to detect an effect, the trial may be stopped.

Baseline comparison

Once the intervention allocation has been revealed, the baseline data (e.g. age, sex, ethnic group, disease grade) are compared between intervention arms to show how successful the allocation process was in producing comparable participants. Differences in baseline characteristics may be due to chance or to biases in the allocation method. If differences are regarded as due to chance, they may be adjusted for by including these factors in a multivariable regression model. If baseline differences may be due to biased allocation, then it will be difficult to interpret whether any differences in outcome are due to the intervention or to bias.

Intervention efficacy

The efficacy of an intervention is calculated as the proportion of outcome that can be prevented by the intervention. This is also known as the 'protective efficacy' or 'preventable fraction' and is the inverse of the attributable fraction (see Chapter 3). **Intervention efficacy** is calculated directly from the relative risk as:

Intervention efficacy = 1 – Relative risk

Intention-to-treat and per-protocol analyses

The primary analysis of an intervention study should be by **intention-to-treat** (ITT). This means that the outcome is compared between study subjects according to the intervention arms to which they were allocated at the start of the study, even if they changed groups, withdrew from the study or were lost to follow-up. Intention-to-treat maintains the original allocation to ensure comparability between intervention arms and reduce confounding (internal validity).

Intention-to-treat avoids selection bias that can arise from different levels of participation during the study. For example, assume that the side-effects of cancer treatment X caused more advanced-stage patients to deteriorate more rapidly and be withdrawn from the study prior to completing treatment. Excluding them from the analysis might result in more severe cases in the comparison arm at the end of the study, mistakenly implying that treatment X was more effective than the control.

The ITT estimate of intervention effect will be closer to what may result in the 'real world', where individuals may not all receive the intervention at the prescribed time points or may not use the interventions as intended. This will provide an estimate that is closer to the effectiveness of the intervention.

However, we might also want to know what the true potential of the intervention might be in an ideal world (e.g. if we were able to improve delivery or compliance). For this reason, a secondary analysis may be carried out **per-protocol**. In per-protocol analysis, only those study participants who receive the intervention according to the pre-defined protocol are included in the analysis. For example, a vaccine trial may specify vaccination of infants at 6–10 weeks, 10–14 weeks, and 14–18 weeks of age. Including infants in the analysis who missed doses or who received doses very late will lead to non-differential misclassification bias and may underestimate the potential of the vaccine.

A per-protocol analysis gives an estimate of the efficacy of the intervention under ideal conditions. It is likely to estimate a larger effect than ITT, because of the dilution of the intervention effect due to the inclusion of non-adherent participants in ITT analyses. However, per-protocol analysis may be subject to bias and confounding if there was a difference in those who complied with the protocol between the comparison arms. It is therefore important to compare ITT and per-protocol analyses to assess the effects of non-compliance on the results.

Meta-analysis

Meta-analysis (see Chapter 5) or a 'pooled analysis' (i.e. grouping individual-level data from several studies) may be used if the effects of the intervention are moderate, if the outcome is relatively rare, or if different epidemiological settings have been studied. This will tend to provide a more reliable and generalizable estimate of effect, and reduce the impact of chance findings from individual trials. Such analyses may be especially useful for measuring rare adverse effects, as most studies would not individually have sufficient statistical power to detect these.

Interpretation

As with all epidemiological studies, results need to be interpreted with caution, considering the roles of chance, bias, and confounding. If the trial has been conducted correctly, with effective allocation and blinding procedures, and has sufficient statistical power, these alternative explanations should not unduly influence the estimated measure of intervention effect. Even if we can infer a causal relationship between exposure to the intervention and frequency of outcome, the findings of an efficacy trial may not be easy to extrapolate to the general population because of the 'artificial' conditions under which they have occurred (e.g. using volunteers, strict eligibility criteria). The results of effectiveness RCTs or non-randomized implementation trials may provide more relevant evidence. Factors such as adverse effects, delivery, cost, and acceptability of the intervention also need to be evaluated before an intervention can be considered for implementation.

✐ Activity 8.5

In The Gambia, infants aged 6–51 weeks who attended a government vaccination facility were screened for eligibility and written parental consent obtained for inclusion in an intervention study. In total, 17,437 children were randomly allocated to receive three doses of either pneumococcal vaccine or a placebo with intervals of at least 25 days between doses (Cutts et al., 2005). They were subsequently monitored for pneumonia over 24 months through attendance at local health facilities and hospital. An independent contractor had labelled vaccine and placebo vials with code numbers using a blocked design and unique study identity numbers. These numbers were subsequently used on health cards, and after the third vaccination had been received, there was no record of the randomization code on the health card.

1. What type of study is this? Be as specific as you can.
2. The results presented included only those children who received the first dose when aged 40–364 days with at least a 25-day interval between doses. What type of analysis is this and which children might have been excluded from the analysis?
3. The incidence rate for first episode of radiological pneumonia was 26.0 per 1000 child-years in infants who received the vaccine and 40.9 per 1000 child-years in infants who received the placebo. Calculate and name an appropriate measure of effect, showing details of your calculations, and interpret your result.
4. The investigators state: 'Efficacy did not vary by age . . .'. Given the information presented in Table 8.2, do you agree with their interpretation? Give reasons for your answer.

Table 8.2 Vaccine efficacy against first episode of invasive pneumococcal disease

Age (months)	% Vaccine efficacy (95% CI)
3–11	93 (54, 100)
12–23	75 (32, 93)
24–29	26 (–339, 89)

Source: Selected data from Cutts et al. (2005).

Conclusion

In this chapter, you have reviewed the key features, advantages, and disadvantages of intervention studies. The experimental nature of this type of study raises many ethical concerns that subsequently drive the specific choice of study design. Intervention studies are generally more complex and costly than other study designs, but are less likely to suffer from bias and confounding. While the double-blind, randomized controlled trial is the gold standard for evaluating most interventions, non-randomized trials are increasingly being employed to assess behavioural and public health interventions.

Additional activities to test your understanding

 Activity 8.6

A multi-centre, double-blind, individually randomized *placebo*-controlled trial in 274 hospitals across 40 countries was undertaken to assess whether early administration of tranexamic acid to 20,211 adult trauma patients with haemorrhage could reduce the risk of death in hospital within 4 weeks of injury. Data were analysed by time from injury to treatment, and showed a relative risk of death due to bleeding of 0.68 (95% CI: 0.5–0.82) if treatment occurred within 1 hour, 0.79 (95% CI: 0.6–0.97) if treatment occurred within 1–3 hours, and 1.44 (95% CI: 1.1–1.84) if treatment occurred ≥3 hours after trauma (Roberts et al., 2011).

1. Interpret these results referring to the study design used, and give your recommendations for the use of tranexamic acid based on these data.
2. In some cases, the injury was not witnessed and the time interval between injury and treatment was estimated. How might this have affected the results?

 Activity 8.7

A trial of a vaccine against Ebola virus disease (EVD) was undertaken during the 2013–2016 outbreak in West Africa. When a case of EVD was identified, all their contacts and contacts of contacts were allocated to a 'cluster'. Clusters were stratified by urban versus rural residence, and by size of cluster (≤20 versus >20 individuals), and were randomly assigned to receive immediate vaccination or delayed vaccination 21 days later. Ebola response teams and laboratory workers were unaware of this allocation. The pre-specified primary outcome was laboratory-confirmed EVD occurring more than 10 days after randomization.

Table 8.3 Results from the EVD vaccine trial

Characteristics	Immediate vaccination	Vaccination after 21 days
Number of clusters	51	47
Number eligible for vaccination	3232	3096
Number vaccinated	2119	2041
Cases of EVD 0–9 days	20	21
Cases of EVD ≥10 days	0	16

Source: Selected data from Henao-Restrepo et al. (2017).

1. Was this a double-blind trial?
2. Why might the investigators have identified clusters of contacts for randomization? [*Note*: Ebola virus is spread by direct contact with body fluids.]
3. Calculate the intention-to-treat vaccine efficacy for days 0–9 post-allocation from Table 8.3, and interpret your result.
4. Calculate the intention-to-treat vaccine efficacy ≥10 days post-allocation from Table 8.3, and interpret your result.
5. Given that not all those eligible were vaccinated, what does this tell us about the effectiveness of this vaccine against EVD?

Activity 8.8

Counselling for Alcohol Problems (CAP) is a brief psychological treatment delivered by lay counsellors to patients with harmful drinking who attend routine primary healthcare settings. Men aged 18–65 years with an alcohol use disorders identification test (AUDIT) score of 12–19 were recruited from 10 primary health centres in India. They were randomly allocated to enhanced usual care (EUC) or EUC combined with CAP within each health centre (Nadkarni et al., 2017). Physicians providing EUC and those assessing outcomes were unaware of the allocation. Primary outcome was remission (AUDIT score <8) at 3 months. Of 190 in the EUC group and 188 in the EUC plus CAP group, 172 and 164 completed the 3-month assessment respectively. There were 44 remissions in the EUC group and 59 in the EUC plus CAP group.

1. What type of intervention study design is this? Be as specific as you can.
2. Calculate the intention-to-treat intervention efficacy from the data provided, and interpret your result.

Feedback on activities in Chapter 8

Feedback on Activity 8.1

There is a clinically proven treatment for this condition, and it may be more appropriate to compare the homeopathic treatment with existing HRT. However, it is unlikely that the homeopathic treatment would be able to achieve the same level of effect, and this may not be a useful comparison.

Given the increased risk of breast cancer, there are reasons to look for an alternative, even if it is less effective. The outcome is not severe, so withholding the best existing treatment would not subject participants to 'additional risks of serious or irreversible harm'. As women are increasingly reluctant to take HRT, it is therefore justifiable to undertake a trial comparing homeopathic treatment to a placebo, if informed consent has been obtained.

Feedback on Activity 8.2

1. This is a multi-centre, open-label (non-blinded), systematically randomized controlled trial. It is 'multi-centre' because subjects were recruited and followed up in several study sites (hospitals). It is 'open-label' because the parents of the infants and those administering the intervention would be aware of whether the infant received an injection or an oral supplement. It is also likely that a clinician recording the outcome would be aware of the child's date of birth and could therefore determine the allocation group. It is 'systematically randomized' because the intervention allocation depends on the day a child was born and is not totally random, but neither is it non-random, because there is usually no choice (either by parents or investigators) about the day a child is born unless it is a scheduled caesarean delivery. Finally, it is 'controlled' because there is a comparison group that receives the existing intervention (not a placebo intervention).

2. You may have identified the following potential limitations.

   - 'Open-label': The study is not blinded, so that parents of infants and those administering the intervention are aware of which intervention is received by an infant. Even the person recording bleeding events may be aware of the allocation, as they will observe the child's date of birth on the medical charts. Knowledge of the intervention allocation may affect a parent's report of adverse events or a clinician's diagnosis of outcome. It would not be justifiable to use an injectable placebo on a newborn, and even if a placebo oral supplement were used, it would not be ethical to withdraw the existing injectable intervention from control arm participants. Therefore, study outcomes would need to be very clearly defined (e.g. amount of bleeding) to reduce subjectivity and potential *information bias*.
   - 'Systematic allocation': The allocation is systematic so that, even if a placebo had been used, investigators could determine the intervention allocation from the child's date of birth. However, children born on odd- or even-numbered days are unlikely to differ in any way and the two groups should still be sufficiently similar to control for any confounding factors. Given that the study is open-label, systematic allocation of the intervention is unlikely to result in any further bias.

- As this is an intervention in newborn children, there may be a high proportion of parents refusing to participate in the study. Alternatively, if injectable vitamin K is routinely given without the need for parental consent, parents may prefer to participate in the study to have a 50% chance of the less invasive oral intervention instead. If parents providing informed consent to participate in the trial differ from those who do not, this may affect our ability to extrapolate these results to the general population.

Feedback on Activity 8.3

1. As the outcome is the number of individuals with at least one fall over a fixed 18-month period, we can calculate the risk of outcome, and therefore the appropriate measure of association is the risk ratio (RR). The RR for group-based exercise was $(76 \div 135)/(87 \div 137) = 0.887$ of 89%, suggesting an 11% reduction in risk of falls. The RR for vision improvement was $(84 \div 139)/(87 \div 137) = 0.952$ or 95%, suggesting a 5% reduction in risk of falls. The RR for home hazard management was $(78 \div 136)/(87 \div 137) = 0.903$ or 90%, suggesting a 10% reduction in risk of falls. This suggests that exercise and home hazard management were equally effective, but vision improvement was less effective. The magnitude of effect here is low for all three interventions, and we do not know the statistical significance of these results.

2. Comparing exercise and vision combined to no intervention, we get $RR = (66 \div 136)/(87 \div 137) = 0.764$ or 76%, so a 24% reduction in risk of falls. Therefore, adding vision improvement to exercise provides an additional 13% protection against the risk of falls compared with exercise alone (11% reduction). You may have compared the combined intervention directly with exercise alone to get $RR = (66 \div 136)/(76 \div 135) = 0.862$ or 86%, indicating a 14% reduction in risk of falls.

3. When developing complex public health interventions, each additional component will have an additional cost. By using a factorial design, we can see the interaction between different interventions, and identify the most effective combination. For example, while vision improvement alone gave a 5% risk reduction, combining it with the exercise intervention gave a 24% risk reduction, which is much greater than we would have estimated by adding the effects of the two individual interventions $(11 + 5 = 16\%)$. The combination of all three interventions gave a $RR = (65 \div 135)/(87 \div 137) = 0.758$ or 76%, indicating a 24% risk reduction, which is the same as exercise plus vision improvement.

Feedback on Activity 8.4

1. As there was already evidence of efficacy (at least in those under 5 years of age), it would not have been ethical to undertake an RCT giving

a placebo to some children. As malaria incidence is seasonal here, it is likely to vary with climate, and therefore historical comparisons would be difficult to interpret. Given that the intervention was being introduced gradually, this would provide an opportunity to undertake a crossover comparison of areas with and without the intervention. Randomizing implementation at the community level would reduce the effect of some confounding factors (e.g. better resourced communities could have earlier implementation).

2. As the introduction of the intervention was progressive over 3 years, the year of implementation would need to be adjusted for in the analysis. The health posts were presumably the unit of cluster randomization, and this would need to be accounted for in the analysis, as children attending the same health posts are likely to have more in common with one another. Children's age and sex may also be confounding factors.

Feedback on Activity 8.5

1. This is a double-blind, randomized placebo-controlled trial of pneumococcal vaccine in infants in The Gambia. It is 'double-blind' because allocation codes and unique identifiers were used so that neither the parents of the infants nor the health personnel assessing the outcomes were aware of the allocation. It is 'randomized' because there was an equal chance of any infant being in either study arm. Finally, it is 'placebo-controlled' because the infants in the comparison group received an identical vaccine that had no active properties against any outcome.

2. This is a per-protocol analysis, as it includes only those who received the intervention as it was originally intended. This analysis would exclude children who were aged less than 6 weeks or more than 52 weeks (1 year) when they received the first dose, those who had less than 25 days between either the first and second or second and third doses, those who did not receive all three doses, and those who may have inadvertently received vaccine instead of placebo or placebo instead of vaccine at any of the three doses. Those who withdrew or died during the study after receiving all doses would still contribute person-time at risk for the period that they were in the study, and would not be excluded from a per-protocol analysis.

3. As this is an intervention study, the appropriate measure of effect would be the vaccine efficacy, calculated as 1 − relative risk. As the reported frequency of outcome is an incidence rate, the appropriate measure of relative risk is the incidence rate ratio = $26.0 \div 40.9 = 0.6357$. Vaccine efficacy is calculated as $1 − 0.6357 = 0.3643$ or 36%, meaning that 36% of episodes of radiological pneumonia in young children in The Gambia can be prevented by vaccination with three doses of the pneumococcal vaccine. [*Note*: You may have calculated it as the preventable

fraction, and this is also correct, as they are the same, although vaccine efficacy is the more specific term in this situation.]

4. You may have stated that you disagree with the authors' interpretation because the estimates of vaccine efficacy are clearly different for each age group. The efficacy appears to decrease substantially with age, and vaccine efficacy is no longer significant in children aged 24–29 months, as the 95% CIs include 0. However, this is an incomplete interpretation of the results.

   The authors' statement is in fact correct. The 95% CIs are relatively wide and overlap between all age groups. This tells us that the estimates of vaccine efficacy are not significantly different between the age groups using a 5% probability cut-off. The difference in the point estimates of vaccine efficacy are likely to be due to a reduced statistical power to detect an effect in older age groups where the sample size may have been too small or the underlying incidence of invasive pneumococcal disease may have been lower.

Feedback on Activity 8.6

1. The protective efficacy of tranexamic acid given within 1 hour of injury is $1 - 0.68 = 0.32$, between 1–3 hours is $1 - 0.79 = 0.21$, and after 3 hours or more is $1 - 1.44 = -0.44$. This means treatment with tranexamic acid can reduce the risk of deaths due to bleeding by 32% if given within 1 hour of injury, by 21% if given within 1–3 hours of injury, and will *increase* the risk of death by 44% if given more than 3 hours after injury.

   The 95% CIs for all three relative risks do not include 1, meaning that these estimates are significant at the 5% level. However, the 95% CIs overlap for treatment within 1 hour and 1–3 hours, suggesting no significant difference between these two periods. Given the size of the study, it is unlikely that these results could be due to chance. The trial was randomized, so it is unlikely that these results could be explained by confounding factors that varied between the study arms. As this was a double-blind trial, there was unlikely to be any information bias that would affect these estimates.

   Given the strength of evidence, the recommendation would be that tranexamic acid should be given as early as possible to bleeding trauma patients. However, tranexamic acid may be harmful for those admitted late (>3 hours) after injury (Roberts et al. 2011).

2. If there were inaccuracies in estimating the time between injury and treatment, this would have led to misclassification of some individuals into the incorrect category of time to treatment. However, this should not have varied between study arms, as the intervention allocation was randomized and blind. Any inaccuracies would therefore have led to *non-differential misclassification* of time-to-treatment, which may have diluted the association between intervention and

outcome. This may have led to an underestimate of the protective efficacy below 3 hours, and an underestimate of the deleterious effect after 3 hours.

Feedback on Activity 8.7

1. No, this was an open-label trial, as both participants and those administering the intervention would have been aware of the allocation. However, those determining the outcome (Ebola response teams and laboratory workers) were unaware of the allocation, so this should have reduced any observer bias.

2. The trial was undertaken during an outbreak of Ebola, so identifying contacts was a way to select individuals at high risk of the outcome. As the intervention was a vaccine, it would have been hard to separate the effects of the individual-level protection from that at the group level, as there may have been some 'herd immunity'. By choosing a cluster-randomized design, the investigators could reduce the effects of contamination between the comparison arms.

3. For intention-to-treat, we use number eligible for vaccination as our denominator. As we have the number of cases but no information on person-time at risk, we can calculate the risk ratio = $(20 \div 3232)/(21 \div 3096) = 0.91$, and vaccine efficacy (VE) = $1 - RR = 1 - 0.91 = 0.09$ or 9%. This indicates little apparent effect of the vaccine within 0–9 days of allocation, as infectious contact may already have occurred prior to vaccination.

4. As in part (3), we can calculate the risk ratio = $(0 \div 3232)/(16 \div 3096) = 0$, so VE = 100%, indicating that this vaccine provides 100% efficacy against EVD after an initial 'washout period' where infectious contact may have preceded vaccination.

5. As only $2119/3232 = 0.66$ or 66% of eligible individuals were vaccinated, a 100% VE suggests that the effectiveness is very high, protecting even those who do not receive it.

Feedback on Activity 8.8

1. This is a multi-centre, individually randomized, open-label controlled trial. Subjects were recruited from 10 primary health centres. They were individually randomized to receive the intervention (CAP) or not. The control arm received an enhanced form of the existing available care, and there was no placebo intervention. It is an open-label trial because participants and those allocating them would have been aware of the allocation, as would those providing the counselling. However, observer bias was reduced since those assessing remission scores were unaware of the allocation.

2. Intention-to-treat requires that we use the original numbers of participants allocated to each group (i.e. 190 EUC and 188 EUC plus CAP). As the outcome is remission at 3 months, and this is a prospective cohort, outcome is measured as a risk, and the appropriate measure of relative risk is the risk ratio. [*Note*: You may have calculated the prevalence ratio, which would give the same answer.] RR = (59 ÷ 188)/ (44 ÷ 190) = 1.355 and intervention efficacy is 1 − RR = 1 − 1.355 = −0.355. Remission is a positive outcome (like survival) and this indicates a 36% increase in remission with the CAP intervention.

SECTION 3

Epidemiology in public health

Prevention strategies 9

Overview

In Sections 1 and 2, you learned how to measure epidemiological associations, assess causality, and gather epidemiological evidence. In Section 3, we discuss how to apply this evidence to different approaches for preventive interventions. In Chapter 9, you will be introduced to the concepts of primary, secondary, and tertiary prevention, and how the shape of the relationship between exposure and outcome influences whether to use a population or high-risk approach to targeting prevention. Screening is a key tool for prevention and we introduce the measures of sensitivity and specificity used to assess the validity of a screening method and predictive values used to assess its utility at an individual level. We review the main criteria for evaluating whether a screening programme should be implemented.

Learning objectives

When you have completed this chapter, you should be able to:

- define strategies in terms of primary, secondary, and tertiary prevention
- distinguish between population and high-risk targeting, and identify the most appropriate strategy for a given situation
- list criteria for assessing the appropriateness of a screening programme
- calculate measures of sensitivity, specificity, and predictive values of a screening method

Levels of prevention

In previous chapters, you learned about conducting rigorous epidemiological research studies and how to evaluate epidemiological results. When there is satisfactory evidence that modification of an exposure can affect the frequency of an outcome, such data can be used to promote good health and prevent or reduce adverse outcomes. Opportunities for preventive intervention relate to the natural development stages of an outcome and are called primary, secondary, and tertiary prevention (see Figure 9.1).

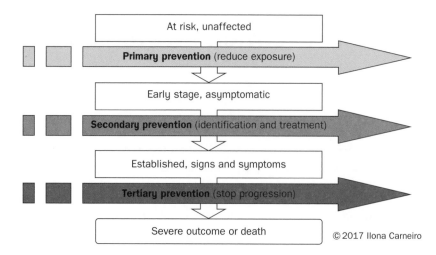

Figure 9.1 The three levels at which interventions for prevention can act, according to progression of outcome

Primary prevention aims to stop an outcome from happening, either by preventing or reducing exposure to a risk factor (e.g. vaccination against an infectious disease, information on risks to encourage behaviour change, such as a reduced weekly alcohol intake). At a population level, this may require societal changes in attitude or new legislation. For example, in Europe, health education campaigns were used to discourage the uptake and continued use of tobacco, then regulation of advertising and increased taxation of tobacco products was introduced, and finally laws were enacted to prohibit smoking in public places and reduce passive smoking (exposure to second-hand tobacco smoke).

Secondary prevention aims to interrupt progression from early to mid-stage of an outcome, mainly by early detection and prompt treatment. An individual may be unaware of having acquired an outcome because they have no symptoms ('**asymptomatic**') or have not noticed the effects ('sub-clinical'). Knowledge of the natural history of an outcome can help development of screening methods to detect the outcome early – screening is a major component of secondary prevention. For example, childhood lead poisoning from house paint or industrial sites can cause seizures, coma, and death. In the USA, blood lead screening is used to identify children at risk while they still have low blood lead levels.

Once the outcome is established and symptomatic, **tertiary prevention** aims to reduce complications or severity by offering appropriate treatments and interventions. For example, renal disease and glaucoma, both complications of uncontrolled diabetes, may be prevented in the diabetic patient if blood glucose levels are successfully regulated using insulin and/or dietary management.

For an outcome such as skin cancer, primary prevention might consist of health promotion campaigns to encourage people to reduce their exposure to the sun (e.g. using sun protection creams and protective clothing). Secondary prevention would focus on detecting and removing skin cancer lesions as soon as they occur to prevent development of invasive melanoma, sentinel lymph node biopsy to assess whether the cancer has spread, and regular check-ups to monitor recurrence. Tertiary prevention would include removal of any affected lymph nodes to prevent further cancer spread, and chemotherapy or radiotherapy to improve **prognosis** if the cancer has already spread.

Activity 9.1

You are responsible for developing a public health strategy to reduce road traffic accident deaths. Describe at which level of prevention each of the following interventions aim to act (*Hint*: describe the progression from exposure to outcome):

1. Vehicle air bags
2. Rapid paramedic care at the crash site
3. Driving speed limits.

Preventive approaches

Differences in individual-level risk factors (relative risk) are likely to be distinct from population-level risk factors (absolute risk). This relates to how exposure varies within and between populations. For example, genetic factors vary more within populations, environmental factors vary more between populations, and behavioural factors are likely to vary between and within populations. This leads to two different approaches to prevention: the individual or 'high-risk' approach and the 'population' approach.

Some preventive measures can only be implemented on a mass scale (e.g. environmental legislation to control air pollution), but for others we can choose whether to act at the individual or population level (e.g. fluoride tablets given to individuals, or fluoridation of the water supply, to prevent tooth decay). The high-risk approach focuses on identifying those at highest risk of an outcome and lowering their exposure to risk factors. The population approach aims to reduce exposure to risk factors in the whole population, often by changing behaviour at a population level.

High-risk approach

The traditional approach to prevention focuses on the individual and reducing their relative risk. For outcomes where the greatest burden is known to be concentrated among high-risk individuals, it may be more appropriate to target high-risk groups rather than the whole population, if we can adequately identify and access those at highest risk.

Other exposures, however, will be more widely distributed throughout a population. While it may be argued that all individuals at risk should have access to interventions that could improve their health, targeting interventions to those at highest risk is often undertaken when an intervention is costly or resources are limited. For example, it would not be cost-effective to provide routine mammograms to women below 30 years of age, given that the main burden of breast cancer is in women over 50 years of age and mammograms are costly.

This approach also fits with society's perception that medical intervention should be focused on those at greatest risk. The general population would be unlikely to consent to testing for sexually transmitted infections (STI) to stop an increasing trend in STI incidence, expecting such screening to be targeted at those who practise 'risky' sexual behaviours (e.g. multiple sexual partners, unprotected sex). Those at greatest risk may also be more likely to comply and therefore benefit from an intervention.

However, risk of outcome and intervention impact are likely to vary within a risk group, and group-level targeting may not enable individuals to make an informed decision about their compliance with an intervention. Labelling individuals as 'high-risk' can cause unnecessary anxiety in healthy people and may even be stigmatizing. Criteria should be standardized to prevent a blurring of categories (e.g. being slightly overweight can merge with being more overweight, which can merge with being labelled 'obese'). This may also shift the burden of responsibility (and 'guilt') to those at highest risk, while failing to recognize the role of external influences (e.g. environment, society) that ultimately affect the wider population.

Another limitation of this approach is that it does not always seek to change the circumstances that encourage exposure to a known risk factor. Vaccination of people at risk of a water-borne disease without efforts to improve the quality of the local water supply, and the use of cholesterol-lowering drugs rather than improving diet, focus on the consequences rather than the cause.

Population approach

The population approach to preventive interventions focuses on reducing the *absolute* risk of an outcome, associated with exposure to a risk factor. For many outcomes, individuals are not simply exposed or unexposed to a risk factor, but may be exposed to varying degrees. Figure 9.2 shows that body mass index (BMI) values are normally distributed. In 1990, very few people were underweight (BMI < 18 kg/m^2), some were obese (BMI ≥ 30 kg/m^2), and the majority were in-between.

Obesity has been associated with an increased risk of cardiovascular disease, hypertension, and diabetes. A high-risk approach to preventive

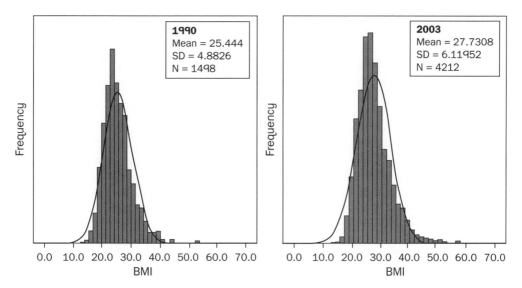

Figure 9.2 Cross-sectional population distribution of adult body mass index (BMI) in Mississippi with superimposed normal distribution curve

Source: Penman and Johnson (2006).

intervention would focus only on those identified as obese. Depending on the relationship between BMI and adverse health outcomes (see below), those who are below the obesity cut-off may be at a lower – but still increased – risk of adverse effects. Individual BMI can change, and we can see how the population BMI distribution has shifted over time. Given this changing exposure with time, interventions aiming to reduce the BMI of the whole population back to 1990 levels might have a greater impact on overall population health than targeted interventions.

Geoffrey Rose advocated that not only do extreme cases require attention, but also the much larger proportion of people with milder features of an outcome. This is because many people exposed to a lower risk of outcome will likely result in more cases than fewer people exposed to a high risk. Therefore, it may make more sense to reduce the population exposure rather than targeting only those at highest risk (for more on this topic, see Fletcher et al., 2013).

✎ Activity 9.2

In the UK, primary prevention of cardiovascular disease (CVD) focuses on identification and management of individuals at high risk of CVD. Studies have shown that an aggressive pharmacological treatment using statins, beta-blockers, ACE-inhibitors, and aspirin can produce a 68% reduction in relative risk of CVD. By targeting the top 10%, 20%, and 30% of middle-aged British men at risk of CVD (based on their total cholesterol and systolic blood pressure), this treatment was predicted to reduce major CVD incidence by 17%, 28%, and 37% respectively (Emberson et al., 2004). By comparison, a 5% reduction in population mean total cholesterol and systolic blood pressure was predicted to reduce major CVD incidence by 26%. Population-wide reductions in mean total cholesterol and blood pressure of 5–15% are consistent with reductions that may be achievable through changes in diet. Based on these data, is it more appropriate to use a high-risk or population approach for primary prevention of CVD in middle-aged British men? Justify your answer.

Prevention paradox

Rose recognized that sometimes 'a measure that brings large benefits to the community offers little to each participating individual' and termed this the '**prevention paradox**' (Rose, 1992). For example, some people may choose to use bicycle helmets to reduce their risk of head injuries. As serious bicycle accidents are rare, most of those who wear a helmet may never benefit from its use, as they will never have an accident. The few helmet-wearing individuals who have a serious accident will reduce their risk of head injury. However, the greatest public health benefit will come from encouraging bicycle helmet use in the whole population, to reduce the overall incidence of bicycle-related head injuries.

Health promotion activities may not motivate individuals if there is little obvious gain for them, so social pressure (e.g. to stop smoking) or economic incentives (e.g. provision of free condoms) may improve compliance. Given the benefit to population health, governments sometimes introduce legislation to achieve population interventions that may otherwise be undermined (e.g. state laws establish vaccination requirements for school children in the USA).

✎ Activity 9.3

Human papilloma virus (HPV) has been identified as a necessary cause of cervical cancer, although it is not a sufficient cause and most of those infected do not develop cervical cancer. A programme of routine vaccination of adolescent girls against HPV is to be conducted in Country X, where the prevalence of HPV among women is 10% and the incidence of cervical cancer is 10 per 100,000 women per year. Is this an example of the 'prevention paradox'? Explain your answer.

Choosing the best approach

As we saw in Chapter 3, the population attributable fraction of an exposure is related to the frequency of that exposure, and reduction in a causal exposure should result in a reduction in the population frequency of the outcome. If we have information on the prevalence of risk factors and a measure of different intervention effects, we can calculate population-attributable fractions to compare the effects of using either a high-risk or population approach to preventive intervention.

There are often benefits to using the two approaches together. For example, in HIV prevention, health education messages on safer sex practices are aimed at the whole population, while sex workers and drug users may be targeted for HIV screening and given improved access to condoms and disposable needles respectively. Choice of strategy will also depend on whether the intervention will be implemented in the community, within hospitals or in a primary healthcare setting. To decide which approach is most appropriate, we need to understand the relationship between exposure and outcome.

Dose–response profiles

Doctors typically classify people as being 'well' or 'unwell', as this helps decision-making about whether to admit a patient, prescribe a drug or perform an operation. However, at a population level, the risk of outcome is likely to vary with changes in the level of exposure. This is known as the 'dose–response' relationship, and Figure 9.3 shows four dose–response profiles proposed by Rose (1992). The shape of the dose–response relationship has an important influence on our choice of prevention approach.

The first relationship represents an exposure that increases without adverse outcome until a 'threshold' level is reached, after which the risk of outcome increases rapidly. For example, an increase in intra-ocular (inside the eye) pressure is not dangerous until it exceeds a certain level. Above this level, the incidence of glaucoma (damage to the optic nerve affecting vision and eventually leading to blindness) rises rapidly. It is therefore desirable to keep intra-ocular pressure under the threshold, but there is no benefit to be gained in further reducing it. In this situation, it would be most appropriate to target preventive interventions to those near the threshold. However, the definition of a threshold level beyond which adverse effects appear is generally derived from population data. At an individual level, some people may experience adverse outcomes below the threshold, while others continue to be healthy above the threshold (e.g. anaemia definitions vary by population).

The second relationship is linear: the greater the exposure, the greater the risk, even at very low exposure levels. For example, there is an increased risk of lung cancer even with the small amounts of tobacco associated with

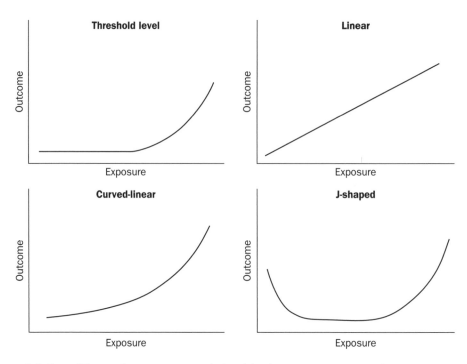

Figure 9.3 Four different dose–response relationships between exposure and outcome
Source: Adapted from Rose (1992).

passive smoking. Shifting the whole population towards lower exposure levels will bring beneficial effects and is the most appropriate public health objective. Health promotion activities and legislation at the population level are the best way to achieve the large change in behaviour necessary to shift population exposure.

The third relationship is 'curved-linear', and may be a more accurate representation of the oversimplified linear relationship. The risk of outcome increases with exposure, but the slope is shallow at lower exposures and increases more rapidly at higher exposures (e.g. maternal age and risk of having a Down's syndrome baby). If most of an outcome is due to those at lower exposure (because few individuals have a high exposure), then it would be appropriate to target the whole population. However, if a large proportion of the outcome occurs in those at higher exposure, then it would be appropriate to target preventive interventions at this high-risk group. For example, in osteoporosis bone mineral density (BMD) is reduced and results in fractures, which can be prevented with appropriate medication. The risk of hip fracture increases gradually with declining BMD until about 700–800 mg/cm^2, below which the risk increases more rapidly. The relative benefit of bone-density X-ray scans depends on the distribution of BMD in the population, and this distribution shifts with age, being greatest in post-menopausal women.

The final 'J-shaped' relationship is the most complex, showing an increased risk of outcome at both low and high exposures. This may sometimes take a 'U-shape', with outcome at high exposure not increasing above that at low exposure. There may also be a range of exposures for which there is no increased risk of outcome, fitting the common belief that 'moderation is good and extremes are bad'. In this situation, there are inherent problems with shifting the entire population too far in either direction, and either a targeted approach or a complex intervention for the whole population is required.

For example, for a given body size, there is a wide range of weight that carries no increased risk of adverse outcome. At the extremes of low weight and high weight, however, there may be associated health hazards. A policy that aims to decrease body weight for the entire population might inadvertently shift some low-weight individuals into the extremely underweight category associated with increased mortality. The health promotion messages therefore need to be more sophisticated and complex, which may make it more difficult to appropriately inform people and encourage healthy behaviour.

Activity 9.4

High alcohol consumption appears to increase the incidence of total and cardiovascular mortality, cardiovascular disease (CVD), stroke, hypertension, diabetes, etc. However, there is evidence that low-to-moderate alcohol consumption is associated with a decrease in CVD compared with those who abstain from alcohol.

1. Which of the dose–response profiles would best describe the relationship between alcohol consumption and CVD?
2. What alcohol-consumption recommendations should be promoted to reduce alcohol-related CVD, and should they be targeted at the individual or population level?

Screening

Screening is a key preventive intervention strategy, enabling early detection and treatment. For example, screening individuals for high blood cholesterol aims to identify those at higher risk of coronary heart disease for targeted health promotion or cholesterol-lowering drug treatment. Once screening identifies individuals at high risk, **diagnosis** may be used to confirm the outcome. Methods of screening and diagnosis include physical examination, blood test, X-ray, and biopsy.

Screening can either use the high-risk ('targeted screening') or population ('mass screening') approach. Targeted screening would measure blood cholesterol only in the relatives of people with familial hypercholesterolaemia (a high cholesterol genetic disorder), whereas mass screening might survey the blood cholesterol of all adults in a population. Screening programmes may be 'systematic' (e.g. all women in the UK aged 25–64 years are reminded to attend for a Papanicolaou cervical smear test every 3 years) or 'opportunistic' (e.g. a clinician measures her patients' blood pressure at every consultation, or offers all sexually active patients under 25 years of age a test for chlamydia infection).

The use of screening assumes that effective interventions are available to reduce risk, or to effectively treat an outcome that is detected sufficiently early. However, issues of cost and limited resources may sometimes lead to controversy and ethical concerns. For example, standard chest X-rays may be used to screen for lung cancer, but they increase exposure to radiation and have not been shown to reduce mortality from lung cancer.

Criteria for screening programmes

The World Health Organization developed criteria in 1968 for assessing the appropriateness of implementing a screening programme (Table 9.1), which continue to guide public health practice. Some of these criteria are context-specific and may differ from the point of view of the individual or population.

Table 9.1 List of 10 WHO criteria for assessing the appropriateness of implementing screening

Focus	Criterion
Treatment	There should be an accepted treatment for those with the condition
Condition	The condition sought should be an important health problem
	The natural history of the condition should be well understood
	There should be a recognizable latent or early symptomatic stage
Method	There should be a suitable test or examination
	The test should be acceptable to the population
Programme	There should be an agreed policy on who to treat
	Facilities for diagnosis and treatment should be available
	Costs (including diagnosis and treatment) should be balanced in relation to healthcare spending
	Screening should be ongoing and not a one-off project

Source: Adapted from Wilson and Jungner (1968).

These criteria have been adapted and new ones proposed, especially with the advent of genetic screening. However, the essential criteria for screening remain:

- the availability of an effective and reliable screening method;
- the availability of an intervention to reduce or improve outcome;

- the safety and acceptability of the test to the individual; and
- that the overall benefits of screening should outweigh any harm to the individual or population.

The relative burden of the condition compared with other health problems should justify the expense of a screening programme in relation to the resources available. Even wealthy societies have finite resources available for health care, and the costs of a screening programme need to be balanced with the cost savings of treating fewer patients identified at a later stage with an advanced outcome. Screening for genetic predisposition may be justified if it affects treatment choice, or can be used for counselling to change other modifiable risk factors.

An outcome that is rare but very serious and easily preventable may still be considered an important health problem. For example, phenylketonuria, a congenitally acquired inability to metabolize the amino acid phenylalanine, is a rare disease. If undetected, it leads to serious mental retardation. A highly sensitive and specific screening test, performed on a blood sample taken from a prick in the heel of a newborn, can identify babies who have this condition. A diet low in phenylalanine can then effectively prevent development of mental retardation in these children. However, with increasing access to affordable genetic testing, the associated costs of counselling and interventions may sometimes outweigh the benefits of screening for rare outcomes.

Operational feasibility

Even if an acceptable test is available and the condition warrants screening, it may not always be feasible to undertake a programme. Screening programmes require systems for identifying and contacting individuals (e.g. practitioner lists, mother and child health clinics, schools) and for ensuring high compliance (e.g. colonoscopy to detect colon cancer is invasive, uncomfortable. and may not be acceptable to sufficient individuals). There are also additional resource requirements, such as the availability of facilities for more extensive diagnostic tests if necessary (e.g. a mammography campaign will result in a greater than usual referral for breast biopsies) and resources for increased treatment (e.g. screening for cholesterol will result in increased demand for cholesterol-lowering drugs).

Evaluating screening

A screening method should ideally be inexpensive, easily administered, and impose minimal discomfort on those to whom it is administered, given that a large proportion of those screened may not be at risk of an adverse outcome. More importantly, the screening method (e.g. ultrasound scan, clinical definition, genetic test) must correctly identify those at risk, and

Table 9.2 Cross-tabulation of true outcome status by screening/diagnostic result

Screening result	True outcome status		Total
	Present	Absent	
Positive	a ('true positives')	b ('false positives')	a + b
Negative	c ('false negatives')	d ('true negatives')	c + d
Total	a + c	b + d	a + b + c + d

this must be evidence-based. The validity of a screening or diagnostic method is its ability to correctly distinguish between individuals with and without the condition of interest (i.e. risk factor, precursor, outcome).

Sensitivity and specificity

The validity of a screening method or diagnostic test is evaluated by calculating its **sensitivity** and **specificity** in terms of detecting an outcome. Sensitivity is the proportion of those who have the outcome who are correctly identified ('true positives'). Specificity is the proportion of those who do not have the outcome who are correctly identified ('true negatives'). An ideal screening method would have both a high sensitivity and high specificity.

The true outcome status of an individual may be determined either by a 'gold standard' diagnostic test (i.e. providing a definitive diagnosis), using the best existing alternative screening method, or by follow-up to observe the outcome. Where the screening method results in a continuous variable (e.g. blood glucose levels for diabetes), this must be categorized into a binomial variable using a defined cut-off based on previous evidence.

In Table 9.2 we compare the distribution of screening method results in relation to true outcome status, and use this to calculate sensitivity and specificity as follows:

$$\text{Sensitivity} = \frac{\text{Number of 'true positives'}}{\text{Number with the outcome}} = \frac{a}{a + c}$$

$$\text{Specificity} = \frac{\text{Number of 'true negatives'}}{\text{Number without the outcome}} = \frac{d}{b + d}$$

The sensitivity and specificity values for a given method are usually not equal, and the relative importance of each depends on the outcome of interest. A low sensitivity means that the screening method results in many 'false negatives' (i.e. it would identify many people *with* the outcome as not having the outcome). A low specificity means that the screening method results in many 'false positives' (i.e. it would identify many people without the outcome as having the outcome).

Higher *sensitivity* is preferred for infectious disease control, to reduce the number of false negatives that could result in continued transmission of the disease. Higher *specificity* is preferred for a screening programme in which subsequent confirmation of an outcome is expensive or invasive (e.g. to avoid performing unnecessary procedures on many false positives), or where a positive result may be stigmatizing.

Predictive values

From an individual perspective, it is more useful to know the 'predictive value' of a screening method. The **positive predictive value** (PPV) is the likelihood of having the outcome based on the test result, while the **negative predictive value** (NPV) is the likelihood of not having the outcome based on the test result. Using the notation in Table 9.2, these are calculated as:

$$\text{Positive predicitive value} = \frac{\text{Number of 'true positives'}}{\text{Number tested positive}} = \frac{a}{a+b}$$

$$\text{Negative predicitive value} = \frac{\text{Number of 'true negatives'}}{\text{Number tested negative}} = \frac{d}{c+d}$$

For example, the PPV of mammography will tell a woman how likely it is that she truly has breast cancer if she has a positive mammogram, while the NPV will tell her how likely it is that she truly does not have breast cancer if she has a negative mammogram.

Predictive values are determined by the sensitivity and specificity of the screening method. The higher the sensitivity, the less likely it is that some-one with a negative result will have the condition, so the higher the NPV of the method. The higher the specificity, the less likely it is that someone with a positive result will not have the outcome, so the higher the PPV of the method.

However, predictive values are also determined by the prevalence of the outcome being screened for. Why? Remember that prevalence is calculated as the number of individuals who have the outcome, divided by the total number sampled. Consider that Table 9.2 has the same format as Table 3.1 (see Chapter 3), and think of the 'screening result' as the 'exposure'. If you compare the formula for prevalence (Chapter 3) with those for PPV and NPV, you will see that these calculate the prevalence of outcome among those individuals 'exposed' and 'unexposed' to a positive screening result respectively. As prevalence decreases, the PPV decreases and the NPV increases, because the overall probability of being positive has declined.

Note that the sensitivity and specificity of a screening method are independent of the prevalence of the condition in the population being screened. This is because sensitivity only relates to those who truly have the condition, while specificity only relates to those who truly do not have the condition. In contrast to predictive values, neither measure considers the frequency (prevalence) of the true condition, and both are calculated from within positives only ($a \div (a + c)$) or negatives only ($d \div (b + d)$).

✎ Activity 9.5

Sepsis is an increasingly common cause of acute illness and death in patients with community and hospital-acquired infections. Early clinical signs are non-specific and there is no gold standard for proof of infection, which may be due to bacteria, fungi, viruses or parasites. Procalcitonin has been investigated as a biomarker for early diagnosis of sepsis in critically ill patients (Wacker et al., 2013). A hypothetical study comparing Procalcitonin to a sepsis diagnosis found 60 true positives, 10 false positives, 40 true negatives, and 5 false negatives.

1. Draw-up a 2 × 2 table to present these results, and calculate the prevalence of sepsis in this study.
2. Calculate the sensitivity, specificity, and positive and negative predictive values from this study, and evaluate whether Procalcitonin is a good marker for early diagnosis of sepsis.
3. In another setting where the prevalence of sepsis was 40%, the positive predictive value of Procalcitonin was 76%. Why would this be, and what would it mean for a critically ill patient with a positive test result?

Before introducing a national screening policy, any additional resource requirements must be planned for. Good quality assurance is essential to ensure correct functioning of a screening programme. Any variation in standards and criteria used to indicate further intervention may result in poor compliance, reducing the proportion of the population likely to benefit. Specialist equipment may be required. Staff may require additional training. Pre- and post-test counselling may be necessary. The incidence of the condition must be estimated to plan for the numbers requiring screening and the subsequent proportion needing further diagnostic tests or expensive treatments. It is unethical to screen if there will be insufficient facilities or effective treatments for those who need them.

Ethical issues

In addition to assessing the validity of a screening method, the ethical consequences of screening must be evaluated at both the individual and population level. The benefits to the individual must be balanced against the costs to society. Similarly, the public health benefit must be balanced against any cost to the individual (e.g. disease reduction or elimination vs any adverse effects of screening).

An unwell person seeking medical help is willing to undergo a medical examination and associated tests in the hope of receiving a definitive diagnosis and appropriate treatment. However, screening is a preventive intervention applied to outwardly healthy people with no symptoms of the outcome. There is an ethical responsibility to provide enough information for individuals to make an informed decision about whether to participate. While many screening methods present no risk, others have the potential to harm the participant (e.g. repeated exposure to X-ray radiation in mammography for breast cancer, or increased risk of miscarriage following an amniocentesis test to identify Down's syndrome pregnancies).

All screening methods will result in false negatives and false positives, either through low sensitivity or specificity, or because of human error. A false positive result can cause unnecessary anxiety while a false negative result can lead to a loss of confidence in a medical intervention or potential loss of life. Someone given a false negative result is provided with a false sense of security and may fail to recognize subsequent symptoms, resulting in poorer outcomes. Even a true positive result may increase anxiety (e.g. genetic testing for Alzheimer's disease), posing a risk to mental health or quality of life, while health and life insurance premiums may also increase.

Measuring effectiveness

The potential effectiveness of a programme to reduce the frequency of a condition can be hard to measure and subject to various biases. **Selection bias** occurs because those who participate in screening programmes often differ from those who do not. Women who are at high risk of breast cancer because of family history may be more likely to attend for mammography. By contrast, women at low risk of cervical cancer appear to be more likely to accept an invitation for a cervical smear test.

Lead-time bias can occur when screening identifies an outcome earlier than it would otherwise have been identified, but has no effect on the outcome (Figure 9.4). Even without medical intervention, it may appear that screening prolongs survival, but this is only a consequence of earlier detection. It increases the length of time the patient knows about their illness, and may lead to greater anxiety and ineffective treatments. This bias can be reduced when evaluating the results of a screening method by using outcome measures other than survival time since diagnosis (e.g. cancer mortality rate rather than 5-year survival rate).

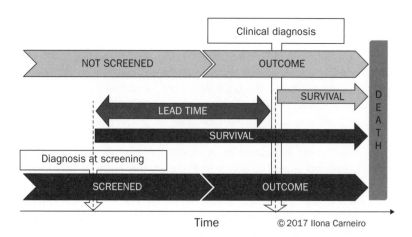

Figure 9.4 Representation of lead-time bias, illustrating how early diagnosis may lead to a longer apparent survival, although the duration of illness is the same

Length-time bias is a form of selection bias and results from screening being more likely to detect outcomes with slow progression (longer asymptomatic or sub-clinical period) than rapid outcomes with a worse **prognosis** (Figure 9.5). For example, slower-growing breast cancer tumours are more likely to be detected by screening prior to the development of symptoms than rapidly growing tumours. However, slower-growing tumours may also be associated with a better survival, leading to an overestimate of screening success. To avoid this bias, effectiveness should be measured for all those with the outcome, and not just those detected through screening. Consider a population of 100 people with cancer: 20 have slower-growing tumours and all are detected by screening, while 80 have faster-growing tumours of which only half (40) are detected by screening before they develop symptoms. If all the slower-growing tumours and none of the faster-growing tumours respond to subsequent treatment, we would calculate the success of screening as 20 ÷ (20 + 40) = 33%. However, the true success should be measured over all those at risk of outcome, as 20 ÷ 100 = 20%.

Screening may also lead to 'over-diagnosis', in which those diagnosed early with sub-clinical disease may have died of other causes before manifesting the outcome. This could result from extreme length-time bias, especially for benign or very slow-growing cancers. An indicator of over-diagnosis after introducing screening would be an increase in early-stage outcome with no effect on late-stage outcome. Through over-diagnosis, individuals may be needlessly turned into patients and exposed to treatments for an outcome that may have never become symptomatic, with associated negative psychological consequences related to such labelling. This may become an increasing problem with genetic screening for outcomes such as breast cancer.

These various biases make it difficult to evaluate screening programmes. Cohort studies comparing the length of survival in those detected through

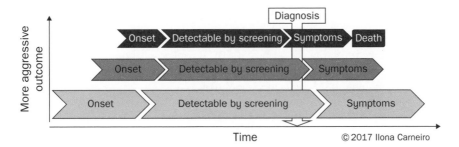

Figure 9.5 Representation of length-time bias, illustrating how variation in length of detectability associated with outcome progression and prognosis provides less opportunity for intervention

screening with those not detected through screening are liable to lead-time and length-time biases. Case-control studies comparing screening history in cases compared with controls are liable to selection and recall biases. Non-randomized trials comparing outcome measures with historical or neighbourhood controls will be liable to selection bias.

The best method for evaluation is therefore the randomized controlled trial (Chapter 8), as most of these biases are removed by random allocation. However, it may not be appropriate to use an RCT for screening if the screening method has already been introduced into a population or if the population perceives the screening as beneficial (even if unproven). It is unethical to undertake a *blind* trial where participants receive placebo screening, as those given a false-negative result from placebo-screening may be less likely to notice symptom development and might delay seeking treatment. If those responsible for subsequent patient care are aware of the trial and subject allocation, this may affect their identification of subsequent symptoms and attribution of cause in the case of death (*observer bias*). There may be a risk of 'contamination' if awareness of a screening programme leads subjects in the control (non-screened) group to seek screening, which may lead to *differential misclassification* of exposure to screening. As many of the conditions that would be screened for are relatively rare, large sample sizes would be necessary to detect a significant effect.

✎ Activity 9.6

A randomized controlled trial of lung cancer screening in male smokers was conducted from 1971 to 1983. The intervention arm was offered a free chest X-ray and sputum cytology every 4 months for 6 years with 75% compliance. The control arm was advised at enrolment to receive the same tests annually. At trial end, 206/4618 and 160/4593 individuals had been diagnosed with lung cancer in the intervention and control arms respectively. Follow-up was extended until 1996 and there was no statistically significant difference in lung cancer mortality between the two arms (Marcus et al., 2000). However, of those diagnosed with lung cancer during the study, the intervention arm showed significantly increased survival since diagnosis.

1. Did the screening intervention work?
2. Discuss the roles of chance, bias, and confounding in these results.

Conclusion

In this chapter, you have learned about primary, secondary, and tertiary levels of prevention that intervene at different stages of outcome development. Public health strategies may be targeted at high-risk groups or applied at a population level, depending on the dose–response relationship, and the distribution of risk and outcome burden in the population. While the population approach is often more effective for public benefit, the 'prevention paradox' may undermine uptake at an individual level, and a combination of the two approaches is often most powerful. Screening is a key strategy in secondary prevention, and you have learned how to evaluate the validity of screening methods (i.e. sensitivity, specificity, and predictive values) and assess the justification for, and effectiveness of, a screening programme.

Feedback on activities in Chapter 9

Feedback on Activity 9.1

As the exposure here is to road traffic crashes and the outcome is mortality, the process of outcome development can be outlined as: (i) road traffic crash, (ii) serious injury, (iii) death. The level of prevention for each intervention can then be explained as follows:

1. Vehicle air bags: Secondary prevention, because air bags act to reduce the severity of injuries resulting from a crash.
2. Rapid paramedic care: Tertiary prevention, because rapid on-site medical care may reduce the risk of death from serious injuries that have already occurred.
3. Driving speed limits: Primary prevention, because speed limits aim to reduce road traffic crashes from occurring in the first place. You may also have said secondary prevention, as a crash is likely to be less severe at lower speeds.

Feedback on Activity 9.2

A similar level of reduction in major CVD incidence can be achieved with a 5% reduction in population mean cholesterol and blood pressure, as with prescribing an aggressive pharmacological treatment to 20% of the population at risk. Identifying those most at risk relies on them accessing formal health care, which may not occur early enough to prevent adverse outcome. A population preventive intervention, including promotion of improved diet, is likely to be less costly than treating 20% of the population at risk, especially when the clinician's time, costs, and potential side-effects of the pharmacological treatments are considered. It is also likely to have other health benefits. Based on these data, it is therefore more appropriate to use a population approach rather than a high-risk approach.

Feedback on Activity 9.3

Yes, this is an example of the prevention paradox, as many girls will receive the intervention but only a small proportion of them will benefit. Most of those to be vaccinated would not have contracted HPV anyway, and most of those who might have contracted HPV would not have developed cervical cancer. Therefore, at an individual level, the reduction in risk is small. However, at a population level, the reduction in risk is great, as HPV-infection is a leading cause of cervical cancer.

Feedback on Activity 9.4

1. This relationship best fits the 'J-shaped' dose–response profile, as the incidence of CVD is highest in those with no or high alcohol consumption, and is lowest in those with low-to-moderate consumption.
2. As this is a complex dose–response relationship, people should be encouraged to reduce their alcohol consumption, but perhaps not to take no alcohol at all. A simple message promoting reduced alcohol consumption could be targeted to those at risk of high consumption. Alternatively, health promotion could be targeted at the whole population, but the message may need to be more sophisticated.

Feedback on Activity 9.5

1. Your table should look like Table 9.3. The prevalence of sepsis in this study is calculated as the total number with sepsis divided by the total number tested = $(60 + 5) \div (60 + 5 + 10 + 40) = 65 \div 115 = 0.565$ or 57%.
2. The sensitivity is true positives divided by the total with sepsis = $60 \div (60 + 5) = 0.923$ or 92%. The specificity is true negatives divided

Table 9.3 Answer to question (1): results of a Procalcitonin test for sepsis diagnosis

	Sepsis	
Procalcitonin	Yes	No
Yes	60	10
No	5	40

by the total without sepsis = 40 ÷ (10 + 40) = 0.800 or 80%. The positive predictive value (PPV) is true positives divided by the total tested positive = 60 ÷ (60 + 10) = 0.857 or 86%. The negative predictive value is true negatives divided by the total tested negative = 40 ÷ (5 + 40) = 0.888 or 89%. Procalcitonin is a good marker for sepsis, as 92% of sepsis cases would be correctly identified enabling appropriate treatment to start promptly and 80% of non-cases would be correctly identified enabling alternative diagnoses to be sought quickly.

3. The PPV was lower because the prevalence of sepsis was lower, and the PPV of a diagnostic test decreases with prevalence of the outcome. A PPV of 76% would mean that a patient with a positive Procalcitonin test would have a 76% probability of having sepsis. This means that there is a 24% (100 − 76 = 24) probability of misdiagnosis in a critically ill patient, resulting in them receiving an incorrect treatment and delaying appropriate treatment.

Feedback on Activity 9.6

1. There was a higher diagnosis of lung cancer in the intervention arm (206/4618 = 4.5%) compared with the control arm (160/4593 = 3.5%), suggesting that detection was higher with enhanced screening, despite a 25% lack of compliance in the intervention arm. Increased survival since diagnosis might indicate a benefit of the intervention, but the lack of a reduction in long-term lung cancer mortality shows that enhanced screening had no effect on the overall outcome.

2. As this is a very large study with a long follow-up, the results are unlikely to be due to chance. Because this is a randomized controlled trial, confounding will have been minimized because randomization of participants should ensure a balance of known and unknown confounders. However, there could be several types of bias here. First, this was an open-label trial and individuals knew which intervention they were receiving, so there may have been misclassification bias if they undertook more- or less-regular screening than they were allocated. Second, the increase in survival time, without an impact on

overall mortality, suggests that there may be lead-time bias, with individuals diagnosed earlier, but no consequent effect on mortality. Third, there may also be length-time bias or over-diagnosis bias, if some of those who were detected early through enhanced screening had less aggressive tumours, and would not have died from them even without diagnosis.

10 | Public health surveillance

Overview

In this chapter, we discuss how routinely collected data can be used to survey the health of populations to quantify health needs and provide an early warning of impending public health problems. Data on process and outcome indicators is also needed to monitor and evaluate treatments, interventions, and public health programmes. The research methods you have learned can be adapted for use under routine conditions, so that public health may continue to be evidence-informed even after research has been completed, helping to inform policy and prioritize practice.

Learning objectives

When you have completed this chapter, you should be able to:

- describe the purpose and types of public health surveillance
- discuss the importance of registries and notifiable outcomes for surveillance
- distinguish process and outcome indicators for monitoring health interventions
- identify methods for evaluating public health programmes
- discuss the role of epidemiological data in informing public health policy and practice

Public health surveillance

Public health surveillance is the monitoring of population health over time to provide timely information on which to base public health decisions, and for the planning, implementation, and evaluation of public health policies and practices. In Chapter 6, you learned about sources of routine data, including civil registration and censuses for demographic data, and health surveys, health facility data, registries, and notifiable outcome reporting for outcome-specific data. We will look at how these sources of data may be used to identify public health problems through routine surveillance, enabling prevention and/or control.

In addition to data on health, it is necessary to collate data on factors known to affect different outcomes (e.g. socio-economic, environmental, behavioural, genetic), as well as data on the health system (e.g. availability and access to care, quality, uptake). A national or sub-national health information system will integrate the collection, analysis, and reporting of data from different sources, to provide evidence for improving health services and ultimately population health.

Routine surveillance

In Chapter 1, you saw an early example of surveillance through John Snow's monitoring of the distribution of cholera-related deaths temporally (i.e. over time) and spatially (i.e. by geographic area). It enabled him to identify a pattern, and to generate and test his hypothesis of drinking water as the source of the epidemic. Regular, systematic, and accurate reporting of health outcomes allows us to determine the usual 'baseline' outcome frequency in a population. If routine data are collected systematically over time, we can study changes in the incidence of an outcome in a population or the impact of a health intervention such as screening or vaccination. An increase in the incidence of measles in a population, for example, can be investigated together with possible explanations (e.g. a decline in vaccination coverage).

Surveillance can detect and verify the emergence of health hazards (e.g. infectious disease outbreaks) or more gradual increases in cause-specific deaths over time that may indicate changes in exposure to a risk factor (e.g. tobacco smoking, HIV). This enables initiation of an appropriate public health response to minimize any adverse impact on the health of a population. A reporting framework is necessary for the systematic collection, analysis, interpretation, and dissemination of health data. While these exist for some infectious and chronic diseases, for many outcomes there is no specific surveillance system in place.

The development of a surveillance system requires clear objectives and the use of strict criteria with which to identify and classify disease. A clear case definition is vital to ensure accurate data are collected and detection is usually based on clinical findings, laboratory results to confirm a diagnosis, and epidemiological data describing the time, place, and type of individuals affected. Standardized reporting methods are essential if authorities are to have confidence in the data collected.

Passive surveillance

Surveillance systems are often passive, relying on data collection at the point of contact with the health service or government agency. Responsibility for reporting is placed on the health service provider, who will routinely collect data on the numbers, basic demographics, and diagnoses of patients seen. Practitioners may also report to registries that centralize data on specific chronic conditions (e.g. cancers) or adverse events (e.g. drug reactions). Passive surveillance also includes the use of certified death data to monitor cause-specific mortality (see Chapter 6).

Many factors can affect data quality, however. Large numbers of people are usually responsible for the collection of surveillance data across many sites. Without the opportunity for specific training, the validity of data may suffer. Feeding back data to the individuals collecting it can motivate them to ensure data are of a high standard. Motivation to record data systematically may also be influenced by the perception of whether the capacity and infrastructure exist to elicit an appropriate public health response.

Health facility data

Public hospitals and clinics generally collect data on outpatient and inpatient attendance, together with basic patient demographics and diagnoses, which is collated and reported to a central body. Health facility data cannot be used to estimate the true incidence of an outcome in the population, because many factors will influence whether an individual attends a health facility. For example, some individuals may seek care from the private, voluntary or informal sectors (e.g. traditional healers, medication sellers) and they would not be included in estimates of incidence calculated from public hospital data. Access to health care also varies with geography and socio-economics.

Health facility data can still be used to monitor the healthcare needs of a population, and as an indicator of what may be occurring in the population, allowing for their biases. For example, an unexpected increase in patients attending with influenza might suggest the start of an epidemic that requires more comprehensive population-based surveillance and health advice.

In low-income settings, where the health services are already overloaded, there may be minimal record-keeping and available data may not be an accurate reflection of the situation. While many effective surveillance systems function around the world, the proportion of outcomes recorded and reported will vary and surveillance is unlikely to capture all cases. Population incidence calculated from routine surveillance is therefore likely to underestimate the true incidence in the community.

Activity 10.1

Rift Valley fever (RVF) is a mosquito-borne viral zoonosis (i.e. it can be transmitted from animals to humans). RVF outbreaks have been reported regularly in Sub-Saharan and North Africa since 2006 and are usually preceded by high rates of abortion among sheep and goats. Most human infections have mild influenza-like symptoms, but RVF can cause more severe symptoms, including haemorrhagic fever and death. In 2011, after several cases were confirmed by laboratory testing, an epidemiological surveillance network for RVF was set up in a low-income African country. What are the main benefits and limitations of using a passive surveillance system that provides reporting forms to village health workers with monthly collection of data?

Outcome registries

Outcome registries collect data on specific outcomes (e.g. type 1 diabetes), together with information on other factors, including basic demographics, patient history, diagnosis, treatment, and health status. Data may come from general practitioners, treatment facilities, hospitals or death certificates. Registries allow the monitoring of individual patients over time and may be used to coordinate recall of patients to attend for regular check-ups and reviews of medication. People may also volunteer to join a registry advertised through patient associations and information websites. Registries can also be used to identify participants for research, such as intervention trials (e.g. the Alzheimer's Prevention Registry), or familial aggregation studies to look for genetic risk factors (e.g. the Breast Cancer Family Registry).

In the UK, the National Congenital Anomaly System (NCAS) was established in 1964 in response to the thalidomide tragedy. Thalidomide was licensed for use by pregnant women as a medication to reduce nausea but was subsequently found to cause limb malformations in the unborn child. The NCAS was set up to detect new hazards and help prevent a similar tragedy. Although the main purpose of the NCAS is surveillance, it also provides valuable birth prevalence data.

Another example comes from Australia's Northern Territory, which reports the highest published incidence of acute rheumatic fever (ARF) in the world among its Aboriginal population. Since recurrent cases of ARF lead to cumulative heart valve damage, ARF is a significant cause of cardiovascular morbidity and mortality for these communities. Since 1997, a rheumatic heart disease control programme has established a computerized registry of all known or suspected cases of ARF or rheumatic heart disease within the region. The registry is used to improve patient care, particularly secondary prevention, by establishing a reminder system for monthly penicillin injections and other clinical follow-up by the primary care system, and to organize and conduct health education programmes.

Registries can be used to monitor outcome incidence, prevalence, and patient survival over time. Analysis of registry data can be used to evaluate the effectiveness of screening programmes, other preventive interventions, treatments, and surgical procedures using cohort study designs. Healthcare providers may also collect information to monitor the quality of care (e.g. treatment waiting times, average length of stay in hospital). By analysing registry data on previous patients, healthcare providers can inform patients and plan, monitor, and improve their services.

✎ Activity 10.2

Data from a national cancer registry showed a threefold increase in the incidence of papillary thyroid carcinoma (PTC) from 1973 to 2006. From 1983, tumour size was recorded and PTC tumours were found to increase by 19%, 12%, 10%, and 12% per year for tumour sizes of ≤1 cm, 1.1–2 cm, 2.1–5 cm, and >5 cm respectively between 1983 and 2006 (Cramer et al., 2010).

1. Based on these data, could the increase in PTC be due to better detection of small tumours?
2. What are the implications of these data for the national health system?

Notifiable outcomes

Many countries have systems in place for monitoring certain notifiable outcomes (e.g. tuberculosis, blood lead levels). Health service providers are legally required to keep detailed records and notify a central public health agency of each case diagnosed (see Figure 10.1). Data are then collated and analysed by public health agencies (e.g. Public Health England, US Centers for Disease Control and Prevention). The initiation of a system for reporting AIDS cases, soon after the syndrome was first described in the USA, provided data that helped to identify high-risk groups and risk factors for the disease, long before its cause was discovered.

The list of notifiable outcomes varies between countries, but the majority are infectious. If the infection is not **endemic** to a country, notification aims to identify importations and stop local transmission. If the infection is endemic, notification enables monitoring for early detection of, and rapid response to, an outbreak.

Notification rates depend primarily on whether an affected individual seeks medical attention. In some communities, healthcare providers may be difficult to access or patients may be unaware of their condition and not seek help. Sometimes, the infrastructure may not exist to record data of sufficient quality or to communicate the data.

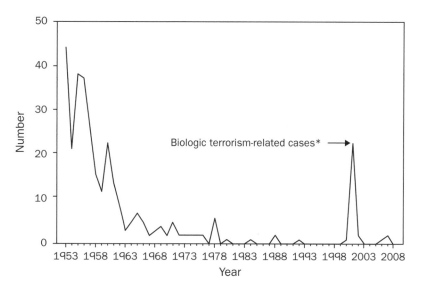

Figure 10.1 Number of cases of anthrax notified by year in the USA, 1953–2008
Source: Centers for Disease Control and Prevention (2010).

Sentinel surveillance

Sentinel surveillance may be necessary when high-quality data are required that cannot be collected through passive surveillance. It involves the identification of health providers and diagnostic facilities with sufficient capacity to collect and analyse the necessary data, and to participate in a reporting network. Designated sentinel sites are selected for their geographic location, disease specialization, and ability to accurately diagnose and provide high-quality data.

Sentinel surveillance may be appropriate when costly diagnostic tests are involved, such as when taking throat-swabs from patients with flu-like symptoms to obtain a laboratory diagnosis of influenza in the UK or monitoring the spread of antimalarial drug resistance across Africa. In low-income countries, this may require an initial investment of appropriate training and resources to develop a functioning network.

Activity 10.3

Antibiotic resistance poses an increasing threat to international public health. In the UK, there has been voluntary reporting of microbiological diagnoses by hospital laboratories, and collection of samples from sentinel laboratories for testing in a national reference laboratory. Data show that the proportion of methicillin-resistant *Staphylococcus aureus* (MRSA) in hospitals increased from 2% in 1990 to 43% in 2001 (Johnson, 2015). As a result, reporting of MRSA by public hospitals became mandatory in 2001. Between 2004 and 2013, the number of MRSA cases reported declined by 56%.

1. Based on the information above, what type of surveillance for antibiotic resistance has been used in the UK?
2. Does the information above suggest any benefit of surveillance for the control of antimicrobial resistance?

Active surveillance

When passive surveillance is unlikely to completely identify cases, surveillance needs to be more proactive, including negative reporting (i.e. reports submitted even when there are no cases). **Active surveillance** may use case-finding techniques (e.g. contact tracing), population surveys or external review of existing clinical records. It is costly and labour-intensive and is not usually used for routine surveillance unless (a) there is a need to monitor the emergence or elimination of a new disease, or (b) when many cases may not be accessing the formal healthcare infrastructure.

Active surveillance is more commonly used for outbreak investigations (see Chapter 6), where results are needed urgently. It can also be used to identify problems with existing passive surveillance, such as the identification of missed AIDS cases through a retrospective review of death certificates and medical records.

Active surveillance may also be used to collate data on the prevalence of known risk factors for adverse health outcomes, such as smoking and alcohol consumption. For example, the US government conducts telephone surveys of more than 400,000 randomly sampled adults each year to obtain nationally representative data through the Behavioral Risk Factor Surveillance System. Similarly, the UK government has a rolling programme of surveillance to assess the diet, nutrient intake, and nutritional status of the population through the National Diet and Nutrition Survey. This enables governments to monitor changes in population behaviours over time, especially related to the burden of chronic disease.

✐ Activity 10.4

Nosocomial (i.e. hospital-acquired) infections are an increasing problem in high-income countries. Hospitals with low rates of nosocomial infection tend to have strong infection-control programmes. Two methods of

hospital surveillance of post-surgery nosocomial infections were compared in several hospitals in a high-income country. Passive surveillance
(clinically diagnosed infections by the surgeon) was found to have
65% sensitivity and 98% specificity when compared with active
surveillance (retrospective review of hospital records and discharge
notes by trained medical personnel). What are the benefits and disadvantages of setting up an active surveillance system for nosocomial
infections in this setting?

Public health response

Data collected through surveillance cannot be used to improve health
unless they are collected, analysed, and transmitted rapidly enough to
enable an appropriate public health response. Surveillance data, trends,
and patterns need to be available to decision-makers to enable evidence-
informed practice.

Early warning systems

Early warning systems collect data on epidemic-prone diseases, to plan,
prepare, and rapidly respond to indicators of outbreaks. This relies on
routine passive surveillance to collect background data, and to identify
patterns and early warning signs of an epidemic or health threat. Case
numbers may be combined with data on other predictors of risk such as
population at risk, or climate and rainfall, to obtain even earlier signals for
preparation.

However, public health agencies need resources and infrastructure to act
rapidly on the information they receive, if they are to successfully stop or
slow the spread of a disease. For example, epidemic-warning systems are
used in the malaria epidemic-prone highlands of Africa. If routine data on
the incidence of clinical malaria cases attending a health facility are
collected and analysed in a timely manner, abnormal patterns can be
identified early, allowing for implementation of preventive measures, such
as indoor residual spraying of houses with insecticide. Previously, delays
inherent in collating paper-based clinic records and summarizing data for
each area resulted in data reaching the malaria control programme too late
to be of use, and clinic staff had no incentive to ensure that data were
rigorously recorded. The introduction of computer databases to enter and
summarize data in real-time, together with appropriate training, improved
the accuracy and utility of this surveillance system (Jones et al., 2008).
Data can now be rapidly fed back to clinic staff and the malaria control
programme, enabling appropriate action.

Similar systems of surveillance are used in emergency settings to identify major outbreaks that may be related to poor living conditions and a breakdown in sanitation and healthcare infrastructure. Monitoring the number of cases of infectious diseases over time (see Chapter 6) can indicate increases that require public health action, such as the isolation of cases to prevent the spread of cholera, or an immunization campaign to reduce measles infection.

Elimination programmes

As more countries move towards the **elimination** of some vaccine-preventable diseases, surveillance takes on a greater role in these programmes. It is essential both as a means of tracking progress towards the goal, and to ensure that any cases are identified early, to prevent outbreaks. Once elimination has been achieved (e.g. measles in the USA in 2000), control programmes enter a maintenance phase focusing on preventing imported cases from re-establishing local transmission, where surveillance is key. For example, surveillance and containment were key to the success of the smallpox eradication programme.

Polio has been eliminated from most parts of the world, but achieving global eradication has proven difficult. The Global Polio Eradication Initiative has worked to strengthen surveillance of polio and reporting systems in low-income countries. As the programme nears its target, the number of cases of paralytic poliomyelitis declines, and detecting circulating wild poliovirus becomes more difficult. While acute poliomyelitis is a notifiable disease, those countries without sufficient infrastructure may rely on reporting of all acute flaccid paralysis cases followed by a laboratory diagnosis. The global programme assesses how effectively a country's surveillance systems are functioning though a network of sentinel sites. Data on cases detected, importations, and local outbreaks are analysed and shared to enable a rapid response using targeted vaccination. In addition to cases of paralysis, surveillance is now supplemented by sampling for the virus in the environment and from stool samples.

✎ Activity 10.5

Measles is a notifiable disease in all WHO European member states, each of which submits regular reports to WHO. The European region had made substantial progress towards the goal of measles elimination in 2015, but an increase in outbreaks was reported to WHO in 2009–2011 (Centers for Disease Control and Prevention, 2011).

1. Why should measles be a notifiable disease in Europe?
2. What is the benefit of regional coordination of surveillance for measles elimination?

Global outbreaks

The World Health Organization (WHO) coordinates several surveillance strategies around the world and aims to strengthen the capacity of countries to conduct effective surveillance. Amid concerns about circulating influenza A virus (H5N1; sometimes called 'avian flu') in the late 1990s, the Global Outbreak Alert and Response Network (GOARN) was initiated in 2000 as a technical collaboration to pool human and technical resources for rapid identification, confirmation, and response to outbreaks of international importance (World Health Organization, 2017b). The subsequent crisis resulting from the Severe Acute Respiratory Syndrome (SARS) epidemic in 2003 in Asia led to an update of the International Health Regulations in 2005 (World Health Organization, 2005). These 'global rules to enhance national, regional, and global public health security', which are legally binding for all member states, came into effect in 2007. The regulations require countries to strengthen their capacities for public health surveillance and response.

The new regulations and network were first tested when an outbreak of influenza A virus (H1N1; sometimes called 'swine flu') was reported to the WHO from Mexico and the USA in April 2009. It was categorized as a 'public health emergency of international concern' (PHEIC) and scientific and epidemiological investigations followed, with unprecedented sharing of information between collaborating institutions (Schuchat et al., 2011), member states, and the WHO. The WHO coordinated surveillance of cases and eventually classified it as a **pandemic** due to outbreaks in countries from different WHO regions. While the extent of the 2009 pandemic was not as great as originally feared, it is difficult to evaluate to what extent this was the result of the early detection, response, and control efforts undertaken in several countries and the efforts coordinated by the WHO.

Since then, WHO has issued PHEIC declarations in response to the resurgence of polio in 2014, the Ebola epidemic in West Africa between 2014 and 2016, and the Zika epidemic in the Americas in 2016. In all situations, the role of surveillance has been vital to recognize the extent of the problem, track geographic spread, and reassure people when the immediate threat was over. While it is challenging to develop surveillance systems during an emergency, especially in countries with poor infrastructure, access to real-time data is key to decision-making under such uncertain conditions. Surveillance data are also important for communicating risk, and the need for often unwelcome control measures, to the public.

Global health

In addition to surveillance at the national level, global trends and national comparisons can also inform public health practice. The Global Health

Observatory collates data on health-related statistics for its 194 WHO member states (World Health Organization, 2017a). A comprehensive analysis of morbidity and mortality outcomes, called the Global Burden of Disease project, is regularly undertaken for all countries using standardized methods and definitions. The disability-adjusted-life-year (DALY) metric was developed in the 1990s, equivalent to one lost year of healthy life, either through premature death or living with a disability of specified severity and duration (Murray and Lopez, 1996). DALYs are primarily used for economic analyses and enable the comparison of the burden of disease across outcomes, risk factors, and geographical regions.

The 2015 Global Burden of Disease study found that age-specific mortality has improved globally since 1980, and the resultant population growth and ageing is placing increased demands on health systems (GBD 2015 Mortality and Causes of Death Collaborators, 2016). It also found that decreases in DALYs due to communicable, neonatal, maternal, and nutritional diseases was offset by increases in DALYs due to non-communicable diseases (GBD 2015 DALYs and HALE Collaborators, 2016). These findings may help to inform public health decision-making on health system investment, prevention efforts, and health policies.

In 2015, the United Nations adopted 17 Sustainable Development Goals (SDGs) as part of a global vision, including good health and well-being for all, to be achieved by 2030 (United Nations, 2015a). As with the Millennium Development Goals (2000–2015) before them, data are needed to monitor progress towards these SDGs, and to evaluate whether the associated 169 targets (e.g. to reduce the global maternal mortality ratio to less than 70 per 100,000 live births) have been reached. In the next two sections, we look at the monitoring and evaluation of public health programmes using descriptive epidemiology.

Monitoring

Monitoring is the term applied to the systematic and routine collection of evidence about the effectiveness of a specific health programme over time, using measureable intermediary and final objectives. Ongoing monitoring enables a programme to adapt and improve, and to reduce disparities in access.

Descriptive epidemiological methods are used to collect data to track the implementation of programmes, measure their progress, and ensure that programmes meet their goals. Monitoring data include process and outcome indicators, such as outcome frequency, associated variables (e.g. anaemia prevalence as an indicator of impact on malaria), and data on adverse events. Data can be collected using cross-sectional or cohort studies, but are more often collected through active or passive surveillance.

Process indicators

Monitoring a public health programme involves measuring how the process is being implemented in relation to pre-specified targets. These 'process indicators' are quantifiable markers of each stage of the process – for example, number of cases detected by a screening programme, number of hospital admissions, or waiting times for surgical interventions. Coverage is a commonly used measure of the proportion of the eligible population that is reached by the intervention (e.g. proportion of children under 12 months old receiving three doses of diphtheria-tetanus-pertussis vaccine, proportion of births attended by a skilled-birth attendant).

For a complex intervention, each step necessary for effective delivery should be monitored. For example, the success of a vaccination pro-gramme will depend on: (a) procurement of a quality-controlled vaccine; (b) delivery of viable vaccine to health centres; (c) sufficient training of health workers on vaccine administration and counselling; (d) availability of viable vaccine, disposable needles and syringes at the time of atten-dance; (e) attendance of the target group (e.g. infants) for vaccination; and finally (f) protection provided by the vaccine. Monitoring may there-fore measure several essential and desirable indicators along a programme's *process pathway*.

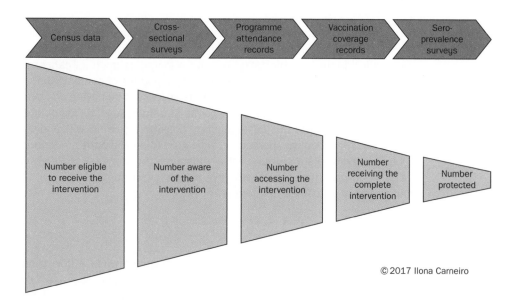

© 2017 Ilona Carneiro

Figure 10.2 Representation of process indicator monitoring to evaluate whether an intervention programme is succeeding

Note: The arrows represent possible sources of data for a vaccination programme, and the pyramid represents the potential for programme failure.

Tracking the process of the intervention allows us to identify any bottlenecks or failures in the system that might be responsible for the differences between efficacy and effectiveness of a public health intervention. Even coverage can be broken down by stages to monitor the process (see Figure 10.2) and identify potential steps in the process that can be targeted to improve the chances of success.

Monitoring may make use of indicators that are collected routinely as part of a country's health information system or indicators introduced as part of a specific health programme. Aspects of programme equity can also be measured by comparing process indicators across groups, for example, using household income quintiles (i.e. dividing the population at risk into five equal-sized groups based on their income) to assess socio-economic equity of access.

To measure coverage or differential access to a health programme, surveys of a representative sample of those at risk can be conducted. For example, routine data from a mother and child clinic may indicate that all infants attending received their measles vaccinations. If we have a good estimate of the number of infants in the community, we can calculate coverage. Otherwise, a household survey may provide more accurate data on *which* households are not sending their children for vaccination – and *why*. This information may be used to improve coverage or equity.

Outcome indicators

During routine implementation of a programme, it may not be possible to monitor the health impact in terms of the outcome of interest, which may be relatively rare (e.g. mortality) or have a long duration (e.g. cancer outcomes). It is therefore necessary to identify indicators of outcome that can be used to assess whether the programme appears to be having any health impacts. If there are sufficient data points (e.g. from several time-points or sub-populations), a correlation analysis of possible indicators with end-point measures may identify appropriate indicators to enable better monitoring. Outcome indicators are often clinical measures that are easy to determine (e.g. blood pressure, cholesterol levels) and known to correlate well with the end-point outcomes of interest.

Adverse events

Data on adverse events should always be collected when a new clinical intervention (e.g. medication, vaccine, medical imaging scan) is being applied to a population. While an intervention must have been demonstrated as safe before it can be implemented, few intervention studies would have sufficient statistical power to detect rare events. Adverse events that may not have been detected during a Phase III trial may become apparent only once an intervention is applied to larger populations, under routine conditions (i.e. poorer compliance or clinical follow-up), and over longer periods of time. Monitoring of adverse events can be undertaken through specially designed Phase IV studies, routine surveillance (e.g. 'pharmacovigilance' for drug-related events) or analysis of healthcare databases (e.g. primary care practice records).

Evaluation

Healthcare evaluation is a broad field, with various components including needs assessment, quality, equity, and cost-effectiveness (for more on this subject, see Tsang and Cromwell, 2017). We will focus on evaluation as a means of measuring a programme's effects and effectiveness. The 'effect' of a programme refers to whether it has achieved delivery of the public health intervention or service, and is usually measured by indicators such as coverage (e.g. proportion of women over 50 attending for a regular mammogram). The 'effectiveness' of a programme refers to whether it has had a measurable public health impact in terms of improving health outcomes, such as the decline in chicken pox (*Varicella zoster*) incidence after the introduction of the varicella vaccine. Programme goals, interim targets to be attained, and methods for assessing effectiveness must be identified beforehand. Evaluation will tend to be periodic, assessing progress against targets at regular intervals to enable any necessary changes to be made.

Plausibility studies (see Chapter 8) may be used to estimate effectiveness by comparing outcome frequency in the population before and after introduction of the programme; comparing a population covered by the programme with a population without access to the programme; or comparing those who did and did not receive a public health intervention. For example, this could include mortality rates among those with short versus long diagnosis-to-treatment intervals, using a pre-defined cut-off. Case-control studies may provide a more rapid means of assessing effectiveness, although they will be subject to different biases (see Chapter 7). For example, cases of *Haemophilous influenzae* type b (Hib) identified from notifiable disease surveillance systems could be compared with community age-matched controls to compare the odds of having received routine infant Hib vaccination (from health records).

Documentation of time-trends following the introduction of a health programme may provide supporting evidence of its effectiveness. However, these 'adequacy evaluations' will not be convincing unless the process pathway is relatively short and simple, the impact is large, and confounding is unlikely (Victora et al., 2004). Process and outcome data must be compared to assess whether any progress can be attributed to the programme. A vaccination programme could not claim responsibility for substantial declines in disease-specific child mortality if insufficient stocks of vaccine had been delivered to vaccination clinics or the number of children receiving the vaccine had been very low.

✎ **Activity 10.6**

This activity is based on the monitoring and evaluation of a malaria intervention programme (Hanson et al., 2008). Pregnant women and children below 5 years of age are high-risk groups for severe malaria outcomes. Insecticide-treated nets (ITNs) provide protection from night-biting mosquitoes to those sleeping under them, and have been proven safe and effective in reducing maternal anaemia and child mortality, particularly in Africa. A programme was established in Tanzania to increase ITN coverage of pregnant women and young children through the delivery of vouchers during the first antenatal care (ANC) visit. Vouchers provided a subsidy (i.e. price reduction) for purchasing an ITN in local shops.

Suppose you are part of a team involved in designing a monitoring and evaluation strategy for this complex intervention.

1. Identify the intermediary processes involved in achieving the programme aims.
2. Which process indicators and methods could be used to monitor how well the programme was functioning and whether it was on track to deliver its outputs?
3. Describe how you would evaluate the effectiveness of the programme after a 5-year period. Identify the primary outcome measure and methods for collecting relevant data.

Epidemiological evidence from research studies is insufficient to advocate for the introduction and continuation of public health interventions. There is great variation in the socio-economic, financial, and environmental contexts within which a programme must operate, leading to distinct programme effects and varying levels of effectiveness in different settings. Without proof that interventions are working, and that they are not causing harm, high uptake and compliance would be unattainable. Evidence that a programme is an efficient (e.g. cost-effective) allocation of often limited resources is also vital for accountability to funders and for planning by policy-makers. Adequate evaluation of public health programmes is essential to ensuring evidence-informed public health practice.

Conclusion

In this chapter, you have learned about how epidemiological methods, rigour, and analysis can be applied to routinely collected data to continually inform public health policy and practice. We reviewed different methods of surveillance from passively collected routine data (e.g. health facility data, outcome registries, notifiable outcomes) to sentinel sites and active surveillance. These systems allow us to identify disease outbreaks and epidemics, monitor time-trends, and identify population-level risk factors for an outcome. Data can be used to plan and prepare for emergencies, prevent re-introductions of eliminated diseases, and stop the global spread of outbreaks. Surveillance methods can also be used to monitor the process and outcome indicators needed to track the progress of public health programmes, including global health goals. Epidemiological surveillance data can be used to evaluate the impact of public health programmes and to provide an evidence base for making informed decisions.

Feedback on activities in Chapter 10

Feedback on Activity 10.1

Routine monitoring by personnel with limited training is unlikely to provide accurate or comparable data. However, this surveillance aims to detect outbreaks, rather than routinely 'monitor' for secular trends or compare populations, and data consistency is therefore not the top priority. The most important issue in this context would be high coverage, which would not be possible with an active surveillance system.

As RVF outbreaks are generally preceded by high rates of abortion among livestock, resident village health workers will be best placed to detect these warning signs. Since most cases have non-specific symptoms, active surveillance would be unable to rely on clinical diagnosis anyway, and laboratory facilities are unlikely to be routinely available.

Collation of monthly reports can be used to 'screen' for areas with increasing numbers of reported influenza-like cases for further investigation. Any reports of cases with more severe symptoms that had not already been notified through the formal healthcare system would identify the local population as being at high risk. A cross-sectional serological survey (i.e. testing antibody levels) could then be conducted.

Feedback on Activity 10.2

1. An unexplained increase in incidence from surveillance data should always be examined for possible changes in diagnostic criteria or detection methods. These data suggest that while there was a much higher rate of increase in the smallest tumours, all tumour sizes showed an increase over the study period. Therefore, better detection of smaller tumours would only partially explain the increase in papillary thyroid carcinoma (PTC). There may have been some other improvement in screening for PTC, or there may have been an increase in the causes of PTC.

2. Regardless of the reasons, a threefold increase in PTC incidence will increase the burden on the health system with respect to increased demands for diagnosis, associated counselling, surgery, and/or radiation therapy. If smaller tumours are more likely to be detected, this may indicate better early-stage diagnosis and improved survival of cases.

Feedback on Activity 10.3

1. A combination of passive surveillance (dependent on voluntary reporting before 2001 and mandatory reporting after 2001) and sentinel surveillance (using selected and quality-controlled facilities) has been used for antimicrobial resistance surveillance in the UK.
2. The information shows that surveillance data highlighted the growing problem of MRSA in 1990–2001, and this had the consequence of increasing the intensity of surveillance for MRSA. We cannot determine what caused the decline in MRSA between 2004 and 2013 from these data. However, given the increasing trend prior to mandatory surveillance, it is likely that mandatory surveillance focused efforts on the problem and played a part in the subsequent reduction of MRSA cases.

Feedback on Activity 10.4

Active surveillance is very costly, taking time and requiring additional staff. However, a sensitivity of 65% means that 100 − 65 = 35% of patients with nosocomial infections were not being identified by the surgeon, i.e. the rate of nosocomial infections was being underestimated. If the surgeons and the hospital are unaware of the magnitude of the problem, it is unlikely it will be resolved.

An active surveillance system would therefore most probably result in better recognition of the burden of nosocomial infections, and subsequent improvements in infection control. As retrospective review does not impact patient care, it may be preferable to set up a sample active surveillance, with retrospective review of a randomly selected proportion of patients as an indicator of the problem.

Feedback on Activity 10.5

1. The only way to eliminate measles – an infectious disease – within the European region is to detect all cases and avert all transmission. By making measles a notifiable disease, symptomatic cases can be identified to enable better detection of sources of infection.
2. As people move across national borders, elimination of an infectious disease can be achieved only by identification of outbreaks and alerting neighbouring countries to the threat. If outbreaks can be identified

quickly, susceptible groups (e.g. migrant populations) can be identified and remedial action can be taken (e.g. mass vaccination campaigns, health promotion to improve routine vaccination coverage).

Feedback on Activity 10.6

1. The intermediary processes can be identified as:

   - Vouchers available in health facilities.
   - Pregnant women attending for routine antenatal care (ANC) visits.
   - Pregnant women receiving a subsidy voucher.
   - Pregnant women seeking to purchase an insecticide-treated net (ITN).
   - ITNs available for purchase with the voucher in the local shops.
   - Pregnant women sleeping under an ITN.
   - Babies or young children co-sleeping under an ITN.

2. Appropriate process indicators for monitoring should correspond to each of the intermediary processes. You may have identified some, or all, of the following.

   - Health facility stock records could be used to document receipt and availability of subsidy vouchers.
   - Health facility records could provide information on the number of women attending for ANC, and demographic data can be used to estimate the number of pregnant women in the population.
   - Pregnant women could be interviewed as they leave the health facility ANC clinic to evaluate what proportion were given a voucher by health facility staff. This is known as an 'exit interview'. These data could also be obtained from a cross-sectional household survey.
   - A household survey might ask about the willingness to purchase a net given that there is some cost to the household. This is a complex issue involving household economics and decision-making powers, and would probably require additional economic and qualitative methods.
   - A structured interview administered to a random sample of shopkeepers could collect data on ITN availability in the local shops, and participation of shops in the voucher programme. This is known as a 'retail audit' and could be undertaken at regular intervals. Additional qualitative data on shopkeeper perceptions of the voucher scheme, collected through semi-structured or in-depth interviews, could identify potential difficulties.
   - Routine programme records on the exchange of vouchers for financial subsidy by shopkeepers could be used to monitor how the process was functioning.
   - A cross-sectional household survey could be used to measure the effects of the programme. The main effects of interest would be the proportion of households with a pregnant woman that own an ITN,

the proportion of pregnant women reporting that they regularly sleep under an ITN, and the proportion of infants or young children reported to regularly sleep under an ITN.

3. While the aim of the programme is 'to increase ITN coverage of pregnant women and young children', its goal is to reduce adverse malaria outcomes in this high-risk target group.

- Child mortality would be hard to measure, and would have to rely on demographic data such as population censuses or representative population surveys, which may not take place within the 5-year time period.
- Maternal anaemia would be the preferred outcome measure, as it could be measured at routine ANC visits. This would not require many additional resources, as training and strengthening of data recording systems would already be implemented in the health facilities and ANC clinics as part of the programme.
- Maternal anaemia is related to low birthweight, which is harder to measure in a low-income country setting, because often a low proportion of births are attended by skilled birth-attendants.
- More direct measures of malaria outcome include outpatient attendance for clinical malaria or hospital admissions for severe malaria. However, these data would be dependent on the quality of data collection at hospitals or health facilities.

Epidemiology in practice 11

Overview

In previous chapters, you have been introduced to the theoretical concepts underlying epidemiology and have reviewed how these are used in research and public health. Here we will review the importance of communicating research and the role of the media. We discuss current public health problems, areas under investigation, and some recent public health emergencies, to demonstrate the key role for epidemiology in society today.

Learning objectives

When you have completed this chapter, you should be able to:

- critique epidemiological research, identifying the key study design issues
- recognize the complexity of epidemiology in practice – specifically issues of ethics, social context, and public engagement
- apply epidemiological concepts to current public health problems
- evaluate a new health threat – from identifying risk factors and causality to interpreting surveillance and assessing proposed methods of control

Evaluating research quality

In the previous chapters, you have seen a variety of examples of epidemiological methods being used to describe health outcomes, to provide evidence of aetiological associations, and to determine the cause of health outcomes. A critical eye can distinguish between real associations, confounding effects, and a weak or biased methodology. In an era of information overload, we must apply this knowledge as a filter to assess the validity of the 'facts' we receive, and to extract evidence-based data to quantify both problems and solutions.

Even those who don't work in health care are now exposed to health information almost daily: from conversations about illness or healthy lifestyle options, to media reports about outbreaks or cancer treatments. As life expectancies increase, individuals look to live healthier and better-quality lives, leading to a constant review of the role of social, environmental, and lifestyle factors in our health. We should encourage a rigorous review of information and evidence-informed decisions in daily life.

Non-scientific reports

There is a deluge of pseudo-scientific information available via social media and the internet. While claims of 'miracle cures' have always existed, non-medical interventions for cancer and HIV, and so-called 'healthy' diet fads are gaining wider public attention, and are often presented as having a scientific basis. Traditional medicines and even home remedies result from accumulated experience and are sometimes proven by scientific testing (e.g. acupuncture, Artemisinin antimalarial treatment), while others are not supported by research (e.g. use of static magnets for chronic pain). There are aspects of physical and mental health that we do not yet understand, or cannot measure, and a lack of scientific proof often merits further investigation.

Headlines to attract readership often result in the misinterpretation or over-simplification of scientific research in the media. Conflicting reports from scientific studies, especially with complex causes for chronic diseases, add to the confusion. There may also be financial interests to encourage or suppress dissemination of certain results. Some key questions to consider when assessing the merit of a reported preventive or risk factor are: the use of rigorous scientific methods (e.g. selection of participants, sample size), repeatability of the findings, and publication in a recognized journal.

Scientific literature

Scientific publications are usually peer-reviewed to ensure a critical appraisal of their methodology and reporting, and potential conflicts of interest need to be clearly stated. One of the main considerations for causality (see Chapter 4) is consistency – the repeatability of a finding – so several studies, in different settings, are often required to confirm an association between an exposure and an outcome.

However, systematic reviews of published research have found that authors are more likely to report statistically significant outcomes and omit non-significant ones, leading to 'publication bias' (Dwan et al., 2013). Therefore, initial studies finding an effect may be published, leading to further research, while those finding no effect may be ignored, ending further research on potentially useful interventions or risk factors of interest. This highlights the need to frame the research question carefully, prepare and adhere to a rigorous protocol, and improve the reporting and publication of research studies.

Implications of poor science

Flawed research can be damaging to scientific progress by diverting limited research funding. Poor medical research can also provide false hope to desperate people or damage the reputation of useful treatments and interventions. One of the most publicized examples is the measles-mumps-rubella (MMR) vaccine controversy.

A report published in the UK in 1998 claimed that MMR vaccination might be associated with the onset of neurodevelopmental disorders such as autism (Wakefield et al., 1998). Despite a sample of only 12 children and selection bias from a self-reported group, the authors emphasized that most parents reported the onset of symptoms after MMR vaccination. Although the scientific community raised concerns, the study received high-profile media coverage, spreading confusion and fear, with many parents refusing to vaccinate their children.

Subsequent investigations found a conflict of interest, unethical practices, and even falsification of data in the original study. Several large epidemiological studies and systematic literature reviews have since shown no association between MMR vaccination and autism, but these took time to conduct, analyse, and disseminate. Unfortunately, reports of an association are more powerful than reports of no association, and public fears surrounding MMR and other childhood vaccinations persist.

 Activity 11.1

1. Describe what Figure 11.1 tells us about MMR vaccine coverage in England between 1997/98 and 2011/12.
2. In 2013, there were large measles outbreaks in the UK, with the highest number of cases in 10–14-year-olds. Suggest a reason for this, referring to Figure 11.1.

Decision-making

When do we have enough evidence to make a public health decision? When a quick result is required, evidence is incomplete or contradictory, or it is too difficult or unethical to undertake relevant research, decision-makers may have to act in the absence of sufficient evidence. By contrast, a lot of research is published, and policy-makers often want local data even when there may be sufficient evidence from other settings. We have seen the need to replicate results to support research findings, especially when the consequences of flawed research can be serious. However, the justification for further research will depend on the amount of variation in previous

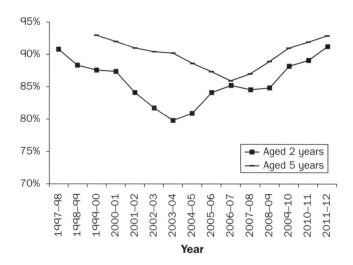

Figure 11.1 Coverage of first-dose MMR in England by year and age group
Source: Ramsay (2013).

findings and the relevance of existing data for the question being asked. The best way to assess existing evidence is to undertake a systematic review.

A systematic review collates relevant published (and increasingly unpublished) research on a topic, such as a treatment or public health intervention, and summarizes the evidence. This involves a thorough search of one or more bibliographic databases, such as PubMed (https://www.ncbi.nlm.nih.gov/pubmed), with clearly defined inclusion criteria. Titles and abstracts are then manually checked for relevance and a final subset of eligible articles is identified. Some systematic reviews then use meta-analysis (see Chapter 5) to combine the results of comparable studies and report a weighted measure of effect. A critical analysis of the selected work aims to provide an objective opinion on the currently available evidence underlying the research topic and to highlight areas that may require further research.

The intention is to use a transparent and well-documented approach to reduce bias, and there are clear guidelines for reporting, including the Preferred Reporting Items for Systematic Reviews and Meta-Analyses (PRISMA) and the handbook from the Cochrane Collaboration. Systematic reviews of preventive interventions, treatments, diagnostic tests, and even prognosis for a given outcome, can all help decision-makers to develop evidence-informed policies.

Evidence into policy and practice

Findings from epidemiological studies and routine data need to be communicated appropriately and rapidly to policy-makers. This requires a dialogue between researchers and policy-makers to shape the research agenda, and produce results that are easily accessible and understandable by end-users. Such scientific 'advocacy' is increasingly important given competing demands for health budgets and overall funding and opposing commercial agendas or social movements. Epidemiological research data are often used successfully to inform public health policy (e.g. national policies on routine childhood vaccination, legislation to reduce exposure to tobacco smoke).

Current issues in public health

In Chapter 1, we saw that considerable progress has been made in the discipline of epidemiology but challenges persist, including: health disparities in access to preventive interventions, diagnosis, and treatment; an increase in chronic diseases and outcomes related to ageing, lifestyles, and pollution; emerging and re-emerging infections related to climate and habitat change; global pandemics and changing health profiles related to international travel and migration. We will look at some of these issues, and apply the knowledge gained from previous chapters to contemporary examples.

Equitable health

Despite the potential of modern medicine to reduce morbidity and mortality, inequity in health outcome and access to health care persists. This is a growing field of research, combining epidemiology with several disciplines, including health economics and social science. There are clearly still many global inequalities in health due to differences in environment, economics, infrastructure, governance, etc. These are often exacerbated by natural disasters and cyclical weather patterns such as the El Niño phenomenon, which affects rainfall patterns and temperatures. While extreme drought in some places leads to malnutrition and famine, heavy rains and floods in other areas are linked to increases in vector-borne and diarrhoeal diseases (World Health Organization, 2016c). Global health equality will benefit from the increased sharing of data and technology, helping governments to prepare contingency plans and undertake surveillance to reduce the impact of such events.

Mobile technologies are helping to improve equity through access to diagnostic tests otherwise unavailable in resource-poor settings, and by helping to disseminate health service information or health promotion messages in remote areas or to those with poor literacy. For example, a smartphone-based assessment of visual function has been developed and validated for use by community healthcare workers (Bastawrous et al., 2015), increasing access to eye health screening, with subsequent prevention or treatment of vision loss for many to whom such health care was previously inaccessible.

At sub-national and community levels, disparities in risk behaviours, exposure to environmental hazards, and the use of preventive services are often associated with socio-economic status but also linked to factors such as gender and ethnicity. This requires the consideration of both horizontal and vertical approaches to improving health equity. Horizontal equity, which requires that people in the same circumstances be treated equally, can be seen in the principle of universal access to health care and preventive interventions. Vertical equity, which requires that people in different circumstances be treated differently in a way that is fair, can be seen in targeted programmes to those most in need once a disparity has been identified.

Health equity must be on both the research and surveillance agendas. Epidemiological methods can contribute to identifying the risk factors for an outcome and monitoring public health programmes to assess their equitability. For example, a comparison of registry data from 53 countries has identified large disparities in childhood leukaemia survival, enabling policy-makers to identify areas of their national health care systems that require improvement (Bonaventure et al., 2017).

✎ Activity 11.2

Screening has been shown to reduce colorectal cancer incidence and mortality, and has been recommended for those aged 50–75 years since 2008 in the USA. Investigators compared the prevalence of reported colorectal screening for the previous years from the national Behavioral Risk Factor Surveillance System telephone surveys. Table 11.1 presents data for the largest ethnic groups.

1. Compare the prevalence of reported screening by ethnic group from the 2004 survey using measures of association to quantify differences, and interpret the findings.
2. Compare the results seen for 2004, 2006, and 2008. What do these results suggest about the equity of colorectal screening by ethnic group?

Table 11.1 Percentage of respondents ≥ 50 years reporting colorectal screening, age-standardized to the 2008 survey population, with 95% confidence intervals (95% CI)

Ethnicity	2004 % (95% CI)	2006 % (95% CI)	2008 % (95% CI)
Non-Hispanic white	58.2 (57.7–58.7)	62.5 (62.0–62.9)	66.2 (65.9–66.5)
Non-Hispanic black	55.3 (53.3–57.2)	58.9 (57.2–60.6)	62.9 (61.5–64.3)
Hispanic	46.0 (43.0–49.0)	47.1 (44.4–49.8)	51.2 (49.2–53.3)

Source: Selected data from Rim et al. (2011).

Chronic diseases

The health burden in many countries is shifting towards chronic diseases, such as cancers, diabetes, and ageing-related outcomes. In addition to lifestyle factors such as smoking and levels of physical activity, nutrition is increasingly the focus of research studies and public health recommendations. For example, the WHO has identified the role of sugars in poor-quality diets, obesity, and the risk of non-communicable diseases (World Health Organization, 2015), and has warned that processed meat consumption increases the risk of colorectal cancer (Bouvard et al., 2015).

While many risk factors for cancer have been identified (e.g. radiation, alcohol, genetics), cancer continues to occur in many people without known risk factors, and vice versa. There are clearly interactions between genes, environmental, and behavioural risk factors, and infections are increasingly implicated in many cancers (Plummer et al., 2016). However, more research is needed to understand the multi-factorial causes of chronic diseases.

One of the largest public health problems today is the epidemic of overweight and obesity, affecting most socio-economic groups in both high- and low-income countries. Obesity is associated with an increased risk of diabetes, cardiovascular disease, hypertension, stroke, and some cancers, and can lead to a poorer quality of life and increased mortality. Many studies on diet, nutrition, and health outcomes have been undertaken, identifying the role of consuming energy-rich and nutrient-poor products. Evidence suggests the obesity epidemic is caused by interactions between diet and physical activity, and there is ongoing health promotion to encourage individual behaviour change.

After years of encouraging the food and beverage industry to self-regulate, some countries have decided to tackle their obesity problem through government regulation and restrictions. For example, many have introduced a tax on sugar-sweetened beverages (SSB), because of evidence that reducing SSB consumption will reduce obesity at an individual level. However, while early studies indicate that these taxes are reducing SSB consumption, evidence of their impact on the prevalence of obesity is not yet available.

✎ Activity 11.3

A meta-analysis of prospective cohort studies compared the association between consumption of sugar-sweetened beverages (SSB), artificially sweetened beverages or fruit juice with type 2 diabetes. The data in Table 11.2 are adjusted for multiple confounders (e.g. family history of diabetes, lifestyle factors) and then additionally for obesity status. Population surveys indicated that 54.4% of the US population consumed SSBs in 2010.

1. Compare the differences seen between the relative risk (RR) unadjusted and adjusted for obesity. What might this suggest?
2. For each beverage category, interpret the final RR adjusted for obesity.
3. The authors attributed 1.8 million excess type 2 diabetes cases to SSBs over a 10-year period in the USA. What assumptions underlie these estimates?
4. Given the information presented, is a tax on SSBs justified to reduce type 2 diabetes?

Table 11.2 Relative risk (RR) and 95% confidence intervals (95% CI) for the association between beverage consumption and type 2 diabetes

Beverage consumed	RR (95% CI) adjusted for multiple variables	RR (95% CI) additionally adjusted for obesity
Sugar-sweetened beverages	1.18 (1.14–1.37)	1.13 (1.06–1.21)
Artificially sweetened beverages	1.25 (1.18–1.33)	1.08 (1.02–1.15)
Fruit juices	1.05 (0.99–1.11)	1.07 (1.01–1.14)

Source: Selected data from Imamura et al. (2015).

It is difficult to tease out the complex associations that exist between nutrition and body mass index, as these are often confounded by differences in physical exercise, stress, and even exposures in childhood and in utero. Large studies on pregnancy and birth cohorts were set up in several European countries in the early 1990s to collect detailed data on exposures in early life. As part of the European Longitudinal Study of Pregnancy and Childhood (ELSPAC), these cohorts and their families have been followed up over decades to see how their life course may affect their health outcomes. Given the interaction of several exposures over our lifetimes, a new area of 'life course epidemiology' has emerged. This aims to investigate the long-term effects and interactions of biological, behavioural, and psychosocial exposures on health outcomes in later life, and even in subsequent generations (Kuh et al., 2003).

Such research may also help us to better understand the causes of dementia, another major public health problem due to growing ageing populations. Genetic studies may help us to understand the molecular and biological basis of neurodegenerative disorders such as Alzheimer's and Parkinson's diseases. It is also possible that increases in risk factors such as physical inactivity and obesity, and resulting cardio-vascular disorders, stroke, and diabetes, may amplify the future burden of dementia.

✎ Activity 11.4

From 1989 to 1994, investigators undertook baseline interviews and assessment for dementia in randomly selected people aged 65 years and older in three areas of England. From 2008 to 2011, the same methods were used to repeat the study. Using age- and sex-specific estimates of prevalence standardized to the 2011 population, 8.3% of the population was estimated to have dementia in the first study compared with 6.5% in the second study.

1. Calculate an appropriate measure of association to compare the frequency of dementia in the second study compared with the first, and interpret your result.
2. What type of epidemiological study is this? Give as much detail as you can.
3. The investigators used logistic regression to adjust for differences in prevalence by age group, sex, and area of residence, and reported an adjusted odds ratio of 0.7 (95% CI: 0.6–0.9, $P = 0.003$). Interpret this finding.
4. Informed written consent was sought from the individuals or their caregivers. The response rate was 80% for the first study period and 56% for the second period. How does this affect interpretation of the study results?
5. A systematic review identified other studies that have shown a reduction in dementia prevalence in higher-income countries. Does this support a causal association between time and prevalence of dementia?

Environmental pollution

With increasing exposure to industrial and environmental pollution, studies on the effect of chronic or accidental exposures are of increasing importance. WHO estimates that 1 in 8 deaths was attributable to exposure to air pollution in 2012, and that more than 90% of the world's population lives in areas where air quality levels are unsafe, making it the largest environmental risk factor (World Health Organization, 2016a). Some of this is caused by household fuel combustion, which alone leads to over 4 million premature deaths per year, in addition to respiratory problems, burns, poisoning, and so on (World Health Organization, 2014).

Another source of environmental risk is electromagnetic fields (EMFs) because of their rapidly increasing use as technology advances. High-frequency EMFs such as X-rays and gamma rays are known to cause cell damage. However, studies on the health risks associated with exposure to low-frequency EMFs (e.g. radio waves, microwaves) have been less clear. Several studies have shown an association between residence near high-voltage power lines and childhood leukaemia. Exposures to EMFs from mobile phones have shown some increased risk of cancer at high levels of long-term use, although their widespread use makes it difficult to undertake conclusive epidemiological studies.

🖉 Activity 11.5

Between April 2014 and October 2015, the residents of Flint, Michigan, were affected by changes in drinking water quality after their water source was switched from the Detroit Water Authority (DWA) to the Flint Water System (FWS). Drinking water can become contaminated by corrosion in lead plumbing, and lead exposure can cause cognitive and developmental disabilities in children and a variety of adverse health effects. Corrosion control was not used at the FWS water treatment plant, and levels of lead in tap water increased over time. In October 2015, the Flint water source was switched back to DWA, and residents were instructed to use filtered tap water for cooking and drinking. All children living at or below the poverty level are routinely tested for blood lead levels (BLL) at 12 and 24 months of age in the state of Michigan, and data on the prevalence of elevated BLLs were available for 2013–2016.

1. Using the information given above, what study design could be used to measure the effect of the water source on blood lead levels? Describe the design in as much detail as you can.
2. Investigators compared elevated BLLs (≥ 5 µg/dL) among children by water source, using logistic regression to adjust for potential confounding factors. They found an odds ratio (OR) of 1.46 (95% CI: 1.06–2.01) for the FWS compared with the original DWA water. Interpret what this result means.
3. The investigators found an OR of 0.75 (95% CI: 0.51–1.12) when comparing elevated BLLs in children after switching back to DWA, compared with the original DWA water. Interpret what this result means for the population of Flint, with regards to environmental lead exposure.

Emerging and re-emerging diseases

Despite the current focus on chronic diseases, infectious diseases still have a prominent role in public health. New infectious diseases are emerging, while others are re-emerging. The main causes are through the appearance of new infectious agents (e.g. HIV), evolution of existing infections (e.g. influenza), transmission to new geographical areas or populations (e.g. West Nile fever), or failure of existing control methods (e.g. drug-resistant tuberculosis).

Conflicts and natural disasters lead to weakened health infrastructure, creating the ideal conditions for public health crises. The most striking example was the importation of cholera to Haiti by Nepalese peacekeepers after the 2010 earthquake. The lack of any immunity in the population was compounded by pre-existing poor health and nutritional status and a lack of safe water and sanitation after the earthquake, which resulted in a severe cholera epidemic that could lead to endemic transmission.

Human behaviour, such as intense farming, keeping domestic pets, hunting, and deforestation, have led to increased threats from 'zoonotic' infections, usually transmitted among animals and only occasionally passed to humans. For example, Ebola virus disease was identified in 1976 with sporadic outbreaks in Sub-Saharan Africa ever since, linked to increased contact with infected wild animals or fruit bats as human populations encroach into forest habitats.

Another growing threat comes from a combination of environmental changes and urbanization, enabling insect vectors to survive for longer and in different habitats. Global climate changes have led to mosquitoes being able to survive long enough to transmit infections, such as malaria, in southern Europe and the USA. Intense urbanization of human populations has given rise to increased breeding of the *Aedes* mosquito, which transmits the dengue, chikungunya, and Zika viruses. Dengue has shifted from occasional severe epidemics prior to 1970 to endemic transmission in over 100 countries, with major outbreaks across the world in 2016.

✏ Activity 11.6

Chikungunya virus emerged in the Caribbean island of Saint Martin at the end of 2013. Figure 11.2 shows weekly cases reported by clinicians and diagnosed at general practitioner clinics. Between 3 and 8 July 2014, all individuals attending a laboratory for any type of biological analysis were offered a serological test to measure previous infection with chikungunya. Those who consented completed a questionnaire including questions on symptoms of chikungunya infection (joint pain and fever) during the previous 6 months. Of 203 individuals tested (93% participation), 42 were seropositive, of which 17 did not report any previous chikungunya-related symptoms.

1. What type of epidemiological data is presented in Figure 11.2?
2. What can you infer from the data presented in Figure 11.2?
3. What type of epidemiological study was undertaken in July 2014?
4. What can you infer from the July laboratory data reported?

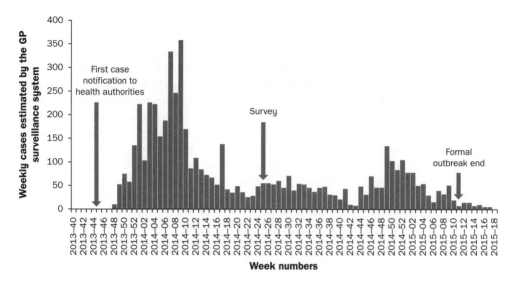

Figure 11.2 Number of weekly incident cases of chikungunya virus on the island of Saint Martin

Source: Gay et al. (2016).

Integrating research and practice

The outbreak of Zika virus in South America in 2015 provides an excellent opportunity to integrate many of the issues that we have covered in this book. The topic is complex and evolving, so we will work through selected information from the timeline provided by the WHO on the origin and spread of Zika (Kindhauser et al., 2016) to consider the identification of the health problem and possible risk factors, the accrual of evidence for causality through epidemiological study, and issues of surveillance.

Zika virus is transmitted by the *Aedes* mosquito and was first identified in a rhesus monkey in Uganda in 1947. Human infections associated with mild illness were reported across Africa and Asia in the subsequent decades. Symptoms are similar to dengue and chikungunya infections, with frequent co-circulation of all three because they are transmitted by *Aedes* mosquitoes. A large outbreak was reported on the Pacific island of Yap in 2007. The virus spread rapidly, with 73% of the 11,250 residents infected, but no deaths or neurological complications reported. In 2013–2014, outbreaks occurred in other Pacific islands, with thousands of suspected cases in French Polynesia.

A new threat

How do we identify a new health threat or an epidemic? Surveillance is the key to early recognition that a problem exists, so the WHO instituted the International Health Regulations (see Chapter 10), requiring every country to conduct surveillance. However, even without good routine surveillance, modern technology allows information to be spread more quickly and we are increasingly aware of health scares that merit further investigation.

In early 2015, more than 7000 cases of patients presented in north-eastern Brazil with symptoms of skin rash, with or without fever. A small percentage were positive for dengue, but were found to be negative for chikungunya, rubella, measles, etc. In May 2015, samples tested positive for Zika virus (Zanluca et al., 2015), demonstrating locally acquired Zika virus in the Americas for the first time. No medications or vaccines against Zika were available in 2015.

✐ Activity 11.7

1. Based on the information above, what would you suggest as the next steps to the Brazilian Ministry of Health?

The WHO Global Outbreak Alert and Response Network provided an opportunity to coordinate national reports and surveillance. In May 2015, the WHO alerted other countries to the Zika outbreak in Brazil. In October, neighbouring Colombia and the Republic of Cabo Verde (with strong ties to Brazil) reported clinical cases with skin rash, and subsequently confirmed the presence of locally acquired Zika virus.

In July 2015, Brazil reported several cases of neurological disorders were associated with a history of Zika, chikungunya or dengue infection. In October 2015, a review of 138 clinical records of patients with a neurological syndrome between March and August found 58 with a previous history of viral infection, of which 32 had symptoms consistent with Zika or dengue infection.

✐ Activity 11.7 (continued)

2. What epidemiological measure can you calculate from these data? Do they show an association between Zika virus and neurological syndromes?

In October 2015, Brazil reported an unusual increase in the incidence of microcephaly (incomplete brain development resulting in a smaller than normal head) in newborns and declared a national public health emergency in November. The WHO subsequently issued an alert to all American countries to monitor and report increases in cases of congenital micro-cephaly and other neurological disorders.

✐ **Activity 11.7 (continued)**

3. Imagine that you are advising the Minister of Health of a country in South America. What would you recommend as priority actions with regard to the apparently separate WHO alerts on: (a) Zika virus infection, and (b) congenital microcephaly and neurological disorders?

Identifying risk factors

In November 2015, Zika virus was found in the amniotic fluid of two pregnant women in Brazil whose foetuses were diagnosed with microcephaly by ultra-sound, and was isolated from the tissue of a baby with microcephaly who died. Retrospective investigations in French Polynesia, reported the same month, documented an increase in congenital neurological malformations during the period of its Zika outbreak, many of which had originally been missed due to pregnancy terminations. In January 2016, there was evi-dence of Zika virus in the brain tissue of two newborns and the placenta of two miscarried foetuses, all with microcephaly, in Brazil. All four women presented with fever and rash during their pregnancies.

In January 2016, El Salvador and Brazil reported unusual increases in Guillain-Barré syndrome (muscle weakness and loss of sensation caused by the immune system attacking the peripheral nervous system). French Polynesia reported retrospective data showing an increase in Guillain-Barré syndrome (GBS) during its Zika outbreak. However, there was also a dengue outbreak at the same time and dengue can also trigger GBS.

✐ **Activity 11.8**

A study was conducted on 42 patients diagnosed with GBS at the central referral hospital in French Polynesia (Cao-Lormeau et al., 2016). Ninety-eight other patients, admitted to or attending for non-febrile illness to the same hospital, were recruited to the study and matched by age (10-year margin), sex, and island of residence to those with GBS. Forty-one patients with GBS tested positive for Zika virus antibodies, indicating recent or previous infection, compared with 35 of the other patients.

1. What type of epidemiological study design is this and was it an appropriate choice? Give reasons for your answers.
2. Calculate an appropriate measure of association between Zika virus and GBS from these data and interpret your answer.
3. The investigators reported a relative risk of 59.7 after adjusting for confounders ($P < 0.001$). Does this prove that Zika virus causes GBS?

Confirming causality

By January 2016, Zika had been identified in several other American countries. On 1 February 2016, the WHO declared the suspected, but scientifically unproven, link between Zika and microcephaly to be a Public Health Emergency of International Concern. However, Cabo Verde reported that its outbreak peaked and declined with no neurological complications detected. The WHO declaration led to a concerted global response and identified a need for research to better understand the relationship between Zika and birth abnormalities.

Activity 11.9

1. Identify the evidence presented so far in favour of, or against, a causal association between Zika virus and birth abnormalities.
2. What further evidence was needed to support causality?
3. What would be an appropriate epidemiological study design to quantify any association between Zika virus infection during pregnancy and birth abnormalities in Brazil in 2016?

In February 2016, the USA reported cases of sexual transmission of Zika virus and Brazil reported a case transmitted by a blood donor. Five more countries reported an increase in cases of GBS associated with increases in Zika virus. Case reports suggested that Zika virus preferentially affects the nervous system.

In March 2016, researchers estimated that the risk of microcephaly in French Polynesia associated with Zika infection during the first trimester might be almost 50 times greater than before the outbreak (Cauchemez et al., 2016). In June, a case study of 1501 live births in Brazil identified a range of birth abnormalities indicating a new congenital syndrome that was 'definitely or probably' related to Zika virus infection (Franca et al., 2016). By the end of 2016, data were available from a cohort study (see Activity 11.10), and preliminary results from a case-control study suggested a 55.5 greater odds of Zika in cases of microcephaly compared with controls (de Araujo et al., 2016).

✐ Activity 11.10

A study enrolled 207 pregnant women in whom a rash had developed within the previous 5 days. All were tested for current Zika virus infection and followed up until pregnancy outcome. Table 11.3 shows selected outcomes according to infection status, and trimester of rash as an indicator of current infection.

1. Calculate appropriate measures of association between Zika infection and reported pregnancy outcomes, and interpret your results.
2. What study limitations can you identify from these data?

Table 11.3 Outcome according to Zika exposure

Variable	Zika-positive	Zika-negative	P-value
Lost to follow-up before pregnancy outcome	9/134	12/73	0.003
Foetal loss (miscarriages or stillbirths)	9/125	4/61	1.00
Adverse outcomes including foetal loss:			
First trimester	11/20	3/4	<0.001
Second trimester	37/72	2/35	<0.001
Third trimester	10/34	2/22	<0.001
Chikungunya infection	3/106	25/60	<0.001

Source: Brasil et al. (2016).

Prevention and control

As more evidence for a congenital Zika syndrome emerged in early 2016 (Rasmussen et al., 2016), the WHO advised pregnant women not to travel to areas with Zika virus outbreaks and for those in Zika-affected areas to delay getting pregnant. People were advised to use mosquito repellents and window screens for personal protection against mosquito bites. Countries at risk of Zika transmission implemented or strengthened vector control used for dengue and chikungunya control. Countries with possible *Aedes* transmission of Zika virus set up surveillance systems to monitor for the infection, neurological cases (Figure 11.3), and birth abnormalities.

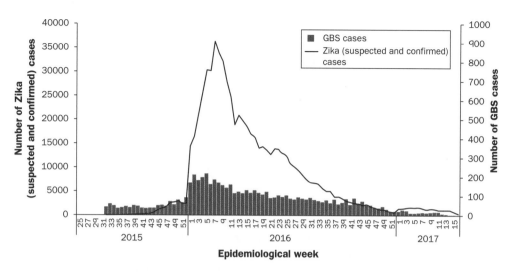

Figure 11.3 Zika and Guillain-Barré syndrome surveillance data reported to the Pan American Health Organization by member countries

Source: Pan American Health Organization (2017).

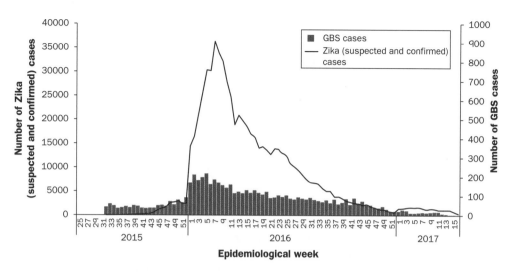

Activity 11.11

1. For each of the following, explain which level of prevention is being acted at to prevent Zika-related birth abnormalities:

   (a) Mosquito nets and/or screening of windows
   (b) Prenatal ultrasound screening for foetal abnormalities
   (c) Provision of contraception.

2. Does Figure 11.3 support an association between Zika virus and GBS? Interpret this surveillance data, using the information presented so far.

Laboratory testing is not always available, and surveillance requires clear case definitions, especially given the similarities of Zika, dengue, and chikungunya cases. In 2016, there were several case definitions in use by different organizations, but no internationally agreed definition.

Activity 11.11 *(continued)*

3. A study compared case definitions with laboratory-confirmed Zika virus in an outbreak in Singapore (Chow et al., 2017). Researchers reported that the Pan American Health Organization (PAHO) case

definition had 49% sensitivity and 76% specificity, while the US Centers for Disease Control (US-CDC) definition had 100% sensitivity and 2% specificity. Interpret what this means, and discuss the advantages and disadvantages of each definition both for local surveillance and for control of the global spread of Zika virus.

Looking ahead

The global spread of Zika virus has raised many interesting issues for public health researchers and practitioners. The description of a new congenital syndrome will require an expansion of the surveillance definition and a longer follow-up of affected children before the full extent of the problem is understood (Costello et al., 2016). It involves a mosquito-borne virus with a wide geographic range of potential transmission, many asymptomatic cases that complicate surveillance and detection, and long-term and severe neurological sequelae that will place a burden on health systems and societies. The threat from Zika virus provides an opportunity for multi-disciplinary collaboration, and the need for international coordination.

Current research efforts are focused on better diagnostic tests, development of vaccines and prophylactic treatments, and a better understanding of the vectors and options for control. Many studies are attempting to understand the risks of congenital Zika syndrome in relation to the severity and timing of infection, the role of confounders and modifying factors (e.g. co-infection with dengue), and the developmental consequences for babies born during the outbreak.

Further research work is also needed to prepare for the impact on the populations affected, with an increased burden of medical care (e.g. care of severely disabled children, diagnosis of hearing, sight, and cognitive problems), psychological and financial costs to the families involved and to society (e.g. lost productivity from adults with neurological complications). Issues of equity will need to be monitored relating to access to preventive interventions (e.g. personal protection from mosquitoes, contraception) and to appropriate health care for those affected. Zika is a complex problem and is likely to be an important public health issue for years to come, at least until we have better diagnostic tests and an effective vaccine, prophylactic treatment or mosquito control.

The future of epidemiology

You have seen how epidemiology continues to be one of the foundations of public health, providing the rigorous evidence base needed to help decision-makers. For those working in health-related fields, the need for epidemiological skills in data collection, analysis, interpretation, and implementation will continue to grow. Epidemiological concepts, such as chance, bias, confounding, and causality, can also help each of us to navigate the growing amounts of information we are inundated with daily.

The challenges of new diseases and complex interactions between exposures will be somewhat balanced by the many opportunities resulting from advances in technology and molecular science. This should result in more 'big data', where information from molecular-level tests (e.g. genetics, different strains of HPV), satellite imagery of the environment (e.g. air pollution), health and lifestyle from wearable technologies (e.g. heart rate, step-counts), and others can be linked together. Data can now be easily stored and shared through cloud-based technologies. High-speed computer processors enable complex multi-level statistical modelling to look at interactions and combined effects of various exposures over time and space.

The importance of collecting high-quality data increases as data access and usage grow. As more agencies and individuals, including policy-makers and the media, have access to descriptive information on the health of populations, its use (and misuse) will increase. We hope that reading this book and working through the activities has given you the incentive and basic tools to collect, analyse, and interpret public health data using effective epidemiological tools.

Conclusion

In this chapter, you have had the opportunity to integrate the skills presented in this book and apply them to real-life public health issues. Throughout the book, we have shifted from research methodology to programme implementation and scientific communication, always considering the concepts of chance, bias, and confounding, in our pursuit of causality. You should now be able to apply epidemiological methods and basic analysis to data from studies or routine monitoring, and interpret your findings to make informed public health decisions.

Feedback on activities in Chapter 11

Feedback on Activity 11.1

1. In 1997–1998, MMR coverage was greater than 90% among 2-year-olds but then dropped gradually over the subsequent years, and more substantially between 2001 and 2003, reaching a low of 80% in 2003–2004. Coverage then appears to increase again, regaining previous coverage levels by 2011–2012. The pattern in 5-year-olds is

similar, showing a lag of 3 years compared with the 2-year-olds. The coverage in 5-year-olds is higher, suggesting delayed MMR vaccination or the effect of catch-up campaigns. [*Note*: The impact of adverse publicity was monitored through surveillance of vaccine coverage and regular surveys of parental knowledge and attitudes.]

2. The children aged 10–14 years in 2013 would have been aged 2 between 2001 and 2005, and aged 5 between 2004 and 2008. This is the cohort with the lowest MMR vaccine coverage (Figure 11.1), and these children were therefore the least protected from measles infection.

Feedback on Activity 11.2

1. In the 2004 survey, the prevalence of reported colorectal screening is highest in non-Hispanic whites at 58.2%, and lowest in Hispanics at 46.0%. There is a significant difference between all three ethnic groups at the $P < 0.05$ level, as the 95% CIs do not overlap. Calculating prevalence ratios (PR) using the non-Hispanic white group as the reference: non-Hispanic blacks have a PR = 55.3 ÷ 58.2 = 0.95 or 5% lower probability of reported colorectal screening; Hispanics have a PR = 46.0 ÷ 58.2 = 0.79 or 21% lower probability of reported colorectal screening. This suggests that Hispanics were much less likely to access colorectal screening in 2004.

2. A comparison of the results from 2004, 2006, and 2008 shows that the reported prevalence of colorectal screening significantly increases over time from 58.2% to 66.2% in non-Hispanic whites, as the 95% CIs do not overlap. Among non-Hispanics blacks there is also a significant increase over time from 55.3% to 62.9%, with only a minor overlap in 95% CIs between 2004 and 2006. Among Hispanics, there was a more gradual increase over time, with an overlap of 95% CIs between 2004 and 2006, and between 2006 and 2008, but a significant increase from 46.0% to 51.2% between 2004 and 2008.

   In 2008, the differences between the ethnic groups remained statistically significant, with no overlap of 95% CIs. The PRs were 62.9 ÷ 66.2 = 0.95 for non-Hispanic blacks and 51.2 ÷ 66.2 = 0.77 for Hispanics. This suggests that while reported colorectal screening increased over time for all three ethnic groups, the ethnic disparity in screening had remained and possibly even increased for the Hispanic group. [*Note*: Reasons for these differences are not evident from the data, but identification of disparities enabled the programme to implement evidence-based interventions to improve coverage in underserved groups.]

Feedback on Activity 11.3

1. After adjusting for obesity status, the relative risk (RR) changed for SSB and especially for artificially sweetened beverage consumption,

suggesting that the association was confounded by obesity status. The RR for fruit juice also changed slightly, suggesting some confounding. (As might be expected, consumers of artificially sweetened beverages tended to be overweight or obese.)

2. All three RR values are greater than 1 and none of the 95% CIs includes 1, suggesting that all three beverage categories are associated with type 2 diabetes after adjusting for several potential confounders. Consumption of SSBs had a 13% greater risk of type 2 diabetes, significant at the $P < 0.05$ level. Consumption of artificially sweetened beverages had an 8% increased risk, and consumption of fruit juices had a 7% increased risk, although the lower 95% CIs were very close to 1, suggesting borderline statistical significance.

3. To attribute cases of type 2 diabetes to SSBs, the authors have assumed a causal association. They have assumed that there are no additional confounders, and that all residual confounding had been adjusted for in their analyses. They have assumed that their estimates of beverage consumption prevalence and type 2 diabetes incidence are correct.

4. This is an example of the prevention paradox. As the RRs are not very high, the individual benefit from cutting out SSBs would not be great. However, the high prevalence of SSB consumption is likely to make this an important risk factor at the population level. Therefore, encouraging a reduction in the consumption of SSBs at the population level should impact the population burden of type 2 diabetes. However, if individuals replace SSBs with artificially sweetened beverages or fruit juice, the potential impact on type 2 diabetes is likely to be diminished. [*Note:* Early evidence suggests that the tax is having the unintended additional consequence of a reduction in artificially sweetened beverage consumption. Also, a reduction in SSB consumption may affect other adverse outcomes such as obesity.]

Feedback on Activity 11.4

1. The outcome measure is prevalence, so an appropriate measure of association would be the prevalence ratio. This is calculated as 6.50 ÷ 8.30 = 0.78, indicating that the prevalence of dementia was 22% lower in the second study compared with the first.

2. This is an ecological study because we are comparing population prevalence rates of dementia, and the exposure is study period. There are no individual-level data involved. [The underlying data come from repeated descriptive cross-sectional surveys, aiming to estimate the prevalence of dementia.]

3. An odds ratio of 0.7 means that the odds of dementia were 30% lower in the second period compared with the first, and this is highly statistically significant, with less than 0.3% probability ($P = 0.003$) of observing this difference by chance. This suggests that the prevalence of dementia declined in this population between 1989–1994 and 2008–2011.

4. The very low response rate for the second study period suggests that there may be some selection bias if there was a systematic difference between those who did and did not respond. For example, those responding and being assessed may have been less likely to have dementia, and those who had dementia may have been less likely to participate. This means that the study may have underestimated the prevalence of dementia in the general population, and that the observed decline in dementia prevalence may have been partially due to selection bias. [Note: The authors found that both very frail and very active individuals were more likely to refuse in the second study. They undertook sensitivity analyses to assess the effect of low response, which confirmed a decline in prevalence.]

5. Additional evidence from other studies fulfils the 'consistency' criteria of Bradford Hill's considerations for causality. However, time alone is not a reasonable causal 'exposure', and other mechanisms need to be identified that would make such a time trend 'plausible'. [Note: The study authors showed that the time-trend was consistent across study areas. Possible mechanisms for this time-trend include large reductions in smoking, and improved management of cardiovascular risk factors in the cohorts studied. However, future generations may suffer from increases in other risk factors.]

Feedback on Activity 11.5

1. The effect of change in water source can be measured by comparing the prevalence of elevated blood lead levels (BLLs) during the different periods of time relating to different water sources. The initial period (January 2013–March 2014) could be considered as the reference 'unexposed' population with water from the DWA, the period April 2014–October 2015 could be considered as the period of 'exposure' to contaminated water from the FWS, and the period November 2015–December 2016 could be considered as an additional post-exposure period with water from the DWA. The prevalence ratios for elevated BLLs between these periods would indicate whether there was an association between water source and BLL, although it would not prove causality. As the comparison is over different time periods, other factors (e.g. season, exposure to other sources of lead such as paint) may confound the association.

2. An odds ratio (OR) of 1.46 means that children had a 46% increased odds of elevated BLLs when they were exposed to water from the FWS compared with water from the DWA. The result is statistically significant at the $P < 0.05$ level, as the 95% CI does not include 1. This suggests that changing the water source to FWS was associated with a nearly 50% increase in the odds of elevated BLLs, if no other temporal changes in lead exposure occurred.

3. An odds ratio of 0.75 would mean that children had a 25% lower odds of elevated BLLs after switching back to the DWA source. However, this result was not statistically significant at the $P < 0.05$ level, as the 95% CI did include 1, and was wide. This suggests that reverting to DWA removed the risk of lead from the water source. However, the slightly lower odds ratio may also indicate that people were following advice to use filtered tap water for cooking and drinking, or even using other sources such as bottled water, and is not sufficient evidence that the environmental risk from the tap water had been removed.

Feedback on Activity 11.6

1. This is passive surveillance data on an outbreak of chikungunya from cases presenting at health facilities and reported by general practitioners.
2. The graph indicates the introduction of a new infection without cases detected prior to week 44 of 2013. It shows three distinct peaks in the number of cases before the outbreak is formally declared over in 2015. The pattern of cases presented suggests that this is a propagated source epidemic (see Chapter 6). However, given that the time-scale spans 18 months (week 44 in 2013 to week 18 in 2015), and that this is a mosquito-borne disease, they may be a result of seasonality, as rainy seasons are related to increased mosquito breeding.
3. A descriptive cross-sectional survey was undertaken in July 2014 to measure the population seroprevalence using a convenience sample of those attending a laboratory.
4. The results suggest that the seroprevalence of chikungunya in July 2014 was $42 \div 203 = 20.69$ or 20.7%. It also suggests that $17 \div 42 = 40.48$ or 40.5% of the chikungunya cases were asymptomatic. While there was a high participation rate, those attending the laboratory may have been different from the general population in some other way (relating to socio-economic access to the laboratory or other illnesses requiring testing), and therefore we cannot be sure that it is a representative sample.

Feedback on Activity 11.7

1. The information known at this point is the appearance of a new viral infection in the country, with symptoms and transmission similar to existing dengue and chikungunya viruses. Sub-national cross-sectional prevalence or seroprevalence surveys would indicate the scale of the Zika burden in the community. It is not especially alarming and existing vector-control measures for the *Aedes* mosquito would probably be continued or boosted in line with normal procedures for an outbreak of dengue or chikungunya. Further steps might involve education of health

personnel as to the existence of this new virus, improved surveillance through laboratory testing of symptomatic cases for Zika, and communication with local scientists to undertake relevant research (e.g. on the vector).

2. The data presented are descriptive, as there is no information on any comparison group of individuals without the outcome, so we cannot calculate any epidemiological measures of association. We can calculate the prevalence of history of viral infection as $58 \div 138 = 0.42$ or 42% among clinical cases with neurological syndromes, and the prevalence of Zika or dengue as $32 \div 138 = 0.23$ or 23% among clinical cases with neurological syndromes. We have no data on Zika virus alone, so these data are insufficient to suggest any epidemiological association.

3. The priority for both issues is to undertake a situational assessment and strengthen surveillance, with clear case definitions in line with those being used by the WHO. If the country did not have any existing vector control or a poor health infrastructure, then help and technical support should be requested from the WHO. You may have suggested something like the following:

   (a) For Zika virus infection, it would be important to communicate with clinicians about the new threat, and to encourage reporting and referral of suspected cases. Laboratories should be given clear guidelines to enable them to test for the Zika virus. Passive surveillance reports of fever cases could be reviewed to identify any increases consistent with an outbreak of any infectious disease, although this may be masked by concurrent outbreaks of dengue or chikungunya. Active case detection could be undertaken in the form of nationwide cross-sectional surveys to measure the prevalence and distribution of Zika virus. Vector-control programmes would need to be implemented or augmented to prevent or control an outbreak. Health messages about the new risk should be communicated to the public, together with information on measures of personal protection (e.g. use of repellents, long clothing, house-screening) and prevention (e.g. removal of *Aedes* mosquito breeding sites such as standing water pots).

   (b) For congenital microcephaly and neurological disorders, it would be important to communicate with clinicians, obstetricians, and hospitals about the WHO alert. Vital registration data could be reviewed if congenital abnormalities are routinely recorded for births. An active review of clinical records (e.g. for referral hospitals) could be undertaken to assess any changes in the incidence of neurological disorders. If such disorders are not already notifiable, this could be implemented to ensure full reporting. However, this would lead to an increase in reports, which would need to be considered when interpreting surveillance data.

Feedback on Activity 11.8

1. This is a matched case-control study analysing the association between Zika virus and GBS. Cases of GBS were identified and matched on age, sex, and island of residence to a convenience sample of hospital-based controls without the outcome. It was the most appropriate choice of design, as the outcome is relatively rare (so a cross-sectional survey would require large numbers) and the exposure was linked to an outbreak, which may not have lasted long enough to undertake a prospective cohort study.

2. As this is a case-control study, the appropriate measure of association is the odds ratio of exposure, as we cannot measure the frequency of the outcome in the population from these data. The odds ratio of having had Zika infection was $(41 \div 1)/(35 \div 63) = 73.8$, suggesting that those who had GBS were 74 times more likely to have been infected with the Zika virus than those who did not have the outcome.

3. The highly significant relative risk (RR) suggests that this association is not due to chance. The cases and controls were matched for age, sex, and island of residence, but we cannot rule out the possibility of residual confounding or confounding by other factors. As this is a case-control study there may be some selection bias, such as those accessing the referral hospital not being representative of the general population. However, the use of hospital controls should have reduced systematic bias between cases and controls. The very large RR from this study supports causality by 'strength of association' between Zika virus and GBS, but it does not prove causality. The reported increases of GBS in French Polynesia, Brazil, and El Salvador also support causality, as they show a 'consistency' of the same relationship.

Feedback on Activity 11.9

1. In 2016, there was no clear evidence to show that prenatal Zika virus infection caused birth abnormalities. Using the Bradford Hill criteria as a framework, we could have identified the following evidence in support of a causal association.

   - Temporality: At a population level, the outbreaks of Zika virus in French Polynesia and Brazil preceded the increase in cases of microcephaly by several months, consistent with infections during pregnancy, although this could also be related to other temporal changes. The January 2016 case study showed that Zika was present in two babies and two foetuses with microcephaly, and that all four women had symptoms consistent with Zika virus during their pregnancies, also supporting temporality.
   - Plausibility: Zika virus was isolated from amniotic fluid, from placenta, and from brain tissue of newborns with microcephaly, showing that

intrauterine transmission of Zika virus can occur. The finding of virus in brain tissue also supports a biological mechanism of action.

- Analogy: Viral infections during early pregnancy (e.g. rubella) have been shown to affect foetal development and cause congenital defects.
- Consistency: An increased number of microcephaly cases were seen in French Polynesia after their Zika outbreak. Although no cases were seen in Yap or Cabo Verde, this may be explained by a low-level risk and small population sizes.
- Coherence: The evidence of trans-placental transmission from case studies, and the increased numbers of microcephaly cases several months after the Zika outbreak, fit together to give a coherent explanation of Zika being responsible for the extra microcephaly cases.
- Strength: No evidence was available.
- Dose–response: No evidence was available.
- Reversibility: No evidence was available.
- Specificity: No evidence was available.

2. Further evidence to support causality would include:

- Strength of association, e.g. a large relative risk of microcephaly babies born to women infected with Zika virus during pregnancy.
- A gradient of effect, e.g. if asymptomatic infections during pregnancy resulted in less severe outcomes than symptomatic infections, this might suggest a dose effect.
- An indication of reversibility, e.g. a decline in microcephaly cases to previous levels after the French Polynesia outbreak had ended.
- Specificity, e.g. if the birth abnormalities seen appear to be clinically similar, and different to defects due to other causes.

3. As this is an emergency outbreak and Zika is a relatively rare outcome, an appropriate study design would be a case-control study. The study would need to be hospital-based to collect blood samples from newborns and mothers, so that any Zika infections could be attributed to the pregnancy period, and avoid misclassification of postpartum infections. The cases and controls could be matched by area of residence and due date, so that they have the same general exposure to Zika, and to reduce potential confounding by other environmental exposures. However, we would not want to over-match (e.g. ethnicity, sex), as this might prevent us from identifying any factors that may modify the association.

A less robust case-control study could recruit cases identified through surveillance, and identify controls in the same community, using reported Zika symptoms during pregnancy (rash and/or fever) as an indicator of exposure. However, this would be prone to selection bias (e.g. there may be a systematic difference between those cases detected by surveillance and community controls), recall bias (e.g. mothers of children with defects may remember symptoms differently to mothers of controls), and misclassification bias because the symptoms of Zika are not very specific and many infections are asymptomatic.

While a prospective cohort study of pregnant women would provide better epidemiological evidence, it would need to be larger and take longer to complete. However, once an association had been shown, it would be the best study design to provide information on risks associated with the timing of exposure. Women could be recruited when attending for prenatal clinics in the affected areas. Blood samples would identify whether the women had already been infected with Zika prior to attendance. Regular blood samples and ultrasound scans from a cohort of initially uninfected women could determine seroconversion, and provide information on the effect of timing of infection and development and severity of birth abnormalities.

Feedback on Activity 11.10

1. As there is no information on the person-time observed, and these are outcomes over a relatively fixed period (gestation), we can calculate the risk of outcome for Zika-infected and uninfected women, and compare them using risk ratios. The risk ratio (RR) of foetal loss was $(9 \div 125)/(4 \div 61) = 1.10$ ($P = 1.00$), suggesting that there was no significant difference in the 'risk' of foetal loss between the two groups. However, there were highly significant differences in the risk of adverse outcomes in each trimester ($P < 0.001$). The RR for the first trimester was $(11 \div 20)/(3 \div 4) = 0.73$, suggesting that Zika-positive women were 27% less likely to have an adverse outcome than Zika-negative women if they had presented with rash in the first trimester. The RR for the second trimester was $(37 \div 72)/(2 \div 35) = 8.99$, suggesting that Zika-positive women were nine times more likely to have an adverse outcome than Zika-negative women if they had presented with rash in the second trimester. Finally, the RR for the third trimester was $(10 \div 34)/(2 \div 22) = 3.24$, suggesting that Zika-positive women were more than three times as likely to have an adverse outcome than Zika-negative women if they had presented with rash in the third trimester. This indicates that Zika infection in the second and third trimesters results in much higher risks of adverse pregnancy outcomes. Although it appears to indicate a protective effect of Zika infection in the first trimester, the numbers are very small.

2. This is a cohort study that recruited pregnant women presenting with rash, so there is selection bias to symptomatic individuals, and the findings cannot be directly extrapolated to the general population of pregnant women. There is a significantly ($P = 0.003$) higher loss to follow-up among Zika-negative women ($12/73 = 16\%$) compared with Zika-positive women ($9/134 = 7\%$), which may suggest another type of

selection bias. If those lost to follow-up are more likely to have suffered an adverse pregnancy outcome, then the measures of association may have been over- or underestimated.

The significantly higher prevalence ($P < 0.001$) of chikungunya infection among Zika-negative women (25/60 = 42%) compared with Zika-positive women (3/106 = 3%) may suggest an alternative explanation for adverse outcomes in the first trimester. The trimester of Zika infection could have been differentially misclassified if women infected earlier in pregnancy presented later with symptoms. Some women who tested negative for current Zika infection may have been asymptomatically infected earlier or later in their pregnancies, again leading to misclassification.

Feedback on Activity 11.11

1. As there are no existing treatments for Zika virus infection, most of the available interventions, such as vector control, will be acting at the primary level to prevent infection from occurring:

   (a) Mosquito screening is acting at the primary level to reduce the risk of being bitten by an infective mosquito and contracting the Zika infection.
   (b) Screening for foetal abnormalities is acting at the secondary level, to either offer affected women the possibility of terminating the pregnancy or prepare psychologically for having a child with abnormalities.
   (c) Contraception is acting at the primary level to prevent a pregnancy that might coincide with Zika infection and lead to birth abnormalities.

2. There is a temporal association between Zika and GBS cases, with an increase seen in both at the start of 2016, and a subsequent decline in cases of both outcomes towards the end of the year. This supports a population-level association between Zika and GBS.

   The low numbers of Zika cases before the end of 2015 might suggest incomplete reporting to the WHO, as Brazil had an ongoing outbreak by this time. The very rapid increase in reported cases of both outcomes at the start of 2016 suggests that there may have been an increase in reporting to the WHO as countries stepped up surveillance in relation to concerns surrounding the association with birth anomalies. There could also have been a lag of surveillance, with some 'catch-up' of cases from the end of 2015 being reported in the first months of 2016. The decline in GBS cases to lower levels in 2017 than at the end of 2015 may suggest incomplete reporting from countries to the WHO. [Note: In fact, not all countries had reported their cases by the time of publication.]

3. A total of 49% of Zika-positive cases and 76% of Zika-negative cases were correctly identified using the PAHO case definition, compared with

100% of Zika-positive cases and only 2% of Zika-negative cases using the US-CDC definition. This means that half of all positive cases will be missed by the PAHO definition, which is not ideal for controlling an outbreak. For South American countries, where Zika is already epidemic, we would want to develop a case-definition with a higher sensitivity, without losing too much specificity.

No positive cases will be missed by the US-CDC definition, but there will be 98% false positives. This is useful when trying to detect importations and prevent an outbreak in the USA, but is highly non-specific and would result in a lot of tests to confirm the diagnosis, which could be unnecessarily distressing for pregnant women and costly for resource-constrained health systems.

Glossary

This is a reference guide to the epidemiological terms used in this book. For further explanation of these terms, use the index to refer to them in the main text. Cross-references to other Glossary terms are shown in *italics*.

Absolute risk See *attributable risk*.

Active surveillance The *surveillance* of an *outcome* by searching for *cases* in the community.

Allocation The distribution of study subjects to *intervention* and *control* arms in an *intervention study*.

Allocation concealment In a *randomized controlled trial*: when the *randomization* schedule for *intervention* allocation is not revealed to the person enrolling subjects, to reduce *selection bias*.

Alternative hypothesis Usually the opposite of the *null hypothesis*, but may indicate the direction of an association.

Analytical study Designed to test a *hypothesis*. Generally, to examine whether an *exposure* is a *risk factor* for an outcome. (Contrast: *descriptive study*)

Ascertainment bias See *information bias*.

Assessment bias See *observer bias*.

Asymptomatic The state of having an *outcome* with no outward *symptoms*.

Attributable fraction (Synonym: *attributable risk percentage*) A measure that calculates the *attributable risk* as a *proportion* of the incidence of *outcome* in those *exposed*, i.e. the proportion of *cases* among those exposed that may be due to the *exposure*, and that could be prevented if the exposure were eliminated completely.

Attributable risk (Synonym: *absolute risk*, *excess risk*, *risk difference*) A measure that calculates the additional frequency of *outcome* in those *exposed* after subtracting the frequency that would have occurred in the absence of *exposure* (i.e. in those *unexposed*). It assumes that the relationship between exposure and outcome is causal, and can be calculated using *prevalence*, *risk* or *incidence rate*.

Attributable risk percentage See *attributable fraction*.

Background risk The frequency of outcome in the unexposed group, therefore also the frequency in the exposed group not attributed to the exposure.

Bias A *systematic* difference from the truth. In epidemiology, this represents a source of error in estimating the association between *exposure* and *outcome*. (See *selection bias*, *information bias*)

Blinding (Synonym: *masking*) Where information about *exposure* or *outcome* is concealed from the participants and/or observers to reduce *information bias*.

Case An individual that meets the *case definition* for having the *outcome* of interest.

Case-control study An *observational study* in which two groups are defined on the basis of their *outcome* status. Those with the outcome are called *cases* and those without the outcome are called *controls*. The level of *exposure* to a *risk factor* is then measured in the two groups and compared. The *odds ratio of exposure* is the only measure of *relative risk* that can be obtained from case-control studies, as there is no measure of the *frequency* of the outcome.

Case definition Criteria for identifying an individual as having the health outcome of interest, which may specify clinical signs and symptoms, diagnostic test results, and time period (e.g. a malaria case as malaria bloodslide positive with reported fever within 48 hours).

Case-fatality rate The *proportion* of cases with an *outcome* that are fatal within a specified period of time. (Note: this is a *proportion* not a *rate*)

Causal pathway The sequence of events leading from an *exposure* to an *outcome*.

Causality The relationship between an *exposure* and a health *outcome*, where the outcome is considered the consequence of the exposure.

Chance The possibility of observing a value or event without reason or predictability. In epidemiology, this is often taken to mean that something is not representative of the reality.

Clinical trial Experiment in clinical research to test new interventions such as vaccines, drugs or medical devices on human participants.

Cluster-randomized trial A *randomized controlled trial* in which groups of individuals (clusters) rather than single individuals are *randomized*, and all individuals within a cluster receive the same *intervention*.

Cohort study (Synonym: *follow-up study*) An *observational study* in which two groups are defined based on their *exposure* to a potential *risk factor*, and are followed up over time to measure the *incidence* of the *outcome*, which is then compared between the groups to give an estimate of *relative risk*. (See *prospective study*, *retrospective study*)

Compliance rate In an *intervention study*: the *proportion* of individuals who cooperate fully with all the study procedures. (Note: this is a *proportion* not a *rate*)

Component cause A factor that contributes to producing an outcome.

Confidence interval The range of values, estimated from a *sample*, within which the 'true' *population* value is likely to be found. A 95% confidence interval is usually presented, meaning that there is a 5% probability that the 'true' *population* value lies outside of this range. It is used to indicate the reliability of the estimated result.

Confounder (Synonym: *confounding variable*) A variable that is associated with both the *exposure* and the *outcome* under study, but is not on the causal pathway between the two. It may provide an alternative explanation for any association observed.

Confounding A situation in which the estimate of association between an *exposure* and an *outcome* is distorted because of the association of the exposure with another factor (see *confounder*) that is also associated with the *outcome*.

Consent See *informed consent*.

Contact An individual that may have interacted with a source of *exposure* such as an infected *case*.

Contamination In an *intervention study*: exposure of the *control* group to the *intervention*, or vice versa.

Control (Case-control) An individual that does not fulfil the *case definition* for the *outcome* of interest. (Contrast: *case*) (Note: this is different to the meaning of *control* in an *intervention* study)

Control (Intervention) A study subject (individual, household, village, etc.) in an *intervention study* who does not receive, and is therefore *not exposed* to, the *intervention* of interest. (Note: this is different to the meaning in a *case-control* study)

Correlation coefficient Usually denoted as '*r*', this measures the strength and direction of a linear association between two variables.

Counterfactual An expression of something that has not happened, but could, would or might have happened, under different conditions.

Cross-sectional study An *observational study* in which information on the *outcome* and *exposure* is measured simultaneously (at one point in time).

Cross-sectional survey A *descriptive* study in which information on the outcome (or exposure) is measured at one point in time.

Crossover trial A *randomized controlled trial* in which each subject acts as its own control by receiving both the *intervention* and *control* at different time points, with a *washout period* in between.

Crude frequency The *frequency* (*prevalence* or *incidence rate*) in the total population, without any adjustment for differences in population structure. (Contrast: *standardized frequency*)

Cumulative incidence See *risk*.

Descriptive study Designed to describe the existing distribution of variables in a *population* without regard to *causal* or other associations. An example would be a *cross-sectional survey* to assess the *prevalence* of anaemia in a population. (Contrast: *analytical study*)

Diagnosis Identification of an *outcome* using rigorous tests or methods.

Differential misclassification Incorrect classification of *exposure* or *outcome* of study subjects because of *information bias*, where this differs between comparison groups. This can lead to over- or under-estimation of a measure of association and may lead to false associations.

Direct standardization See *standardization*.

Ecological bias (Synonym: *ecological fallacy*)

Ecological fallacy (Synonym: *ecological bias*) The misguided idea that a group-level association from an *ecological study* can be applied at the individual level.

Ecological study An *observational study* in which the units of analysis are populations or groups of people rather than individuals. (See *ecological fallacy*)

Effect modification (Synonym: *interaction*) Variation in the effect of the *exposure* on an *outcome* across values of another factor (*effect modifier*). It can be detected by *stratification* during analysis and may be adjusted for with *statistical modelling*.

Effect modifier Factor across whose categories the effect of an *exposure* on outcome may vary. (See *effect modification*)

Effectiveness The extent to which an *intervention* produces an improvement in a health *outcome* when it is applied through a routine delivery system. (Contrast: *efficacy*)

Efficacy The extent to which an *intervention* produces an improvement in a health *outcome* under ideal trial conditions. (Contrast: *effectiveness*)

Elimination The total removal of an *outcome* (usually by removal of the *exposure*) from a country or region. (Contrast: *eradication*)

Endemic The maintenance of an infection in a defined *population* without external introduction.

Epidemic The increase in the *frequency* of an *outcome* that is significantly more than would normally be expected.

Equivalence trial A *randomized-controlled trial* which aims to determine that two interventions are similar to each other.

Eradication The total removal of an *outcome* (usually by removal of the *exposure*) from the entire world. (Contrast: *elimination*)

Excess risk See *attributable risk*.

Exclusion criteria Characteristics defining which individuals may not be included in a study. (Contrast: *inclusion criteria*)

Exposed Those subjects who have experienced or possess (e.g. genetic or physical characteristics) the *risk factor* of interest.

Exposure Synonymous with *risk factor*, or the act of being exposed to a potential risk or *protective factor*.

External validity The extent to which the results of a study can be generalized to the population that the study sample was meant to represent. (Contrast: *internal validity*)

Factorial trial A *randomized controlled trial* in which two or more *interventions* are compared individually and in combination against a *control* comparison group.

Follow-up Prospective observation over time of an individual, group or initially defined population whose relevant characteristics have been assessed to observe changes in *exposures* or *outcomes*.

Frequency A measure of the number of occurrences of an outcome per *population* (see *prevalence*) or per unit time (see *incidence*).

General population The wider population to whom the results of analytical epidemiological studies are to be applied. For example, the 'general population of India' refers to all individuals living in India. (Contrast: *sample population*, *target population*)

Hypothesis A supposition phrased in such a way as to allow it to be tested and confirmed or refuted.

Incidence The number of new *cases* of an *outcome* that develop in a defined *population* of individuals at risk during a specified period. It can be measured as *risk, odds* or *incidence rate.* (See *null hypothesis*)

Incidence rate The number of new *cases* of an *outcome* that develop in a defined *population* of individuals at risk during a specified period of time, divided by the total *person-time at risk.*

Incidence rate ratio (Synonym: *rate ratio*) A measure of *relative risk.* Calculated as the *incidence rate* of *outcome* in those exposed, divided by the incidence rate of outcome in those unexposed.

Inclusion criteria Characteristics defining which individuals may be included in a study. (Contrast: *exclusion criteria*)

Indirect standardization See *standardization.*

Information bias (Synonym: *ascertainment bias*) Error due to *systematic* differences in the classification *exposure* or *outcome* status of study participants. (See *measurement bias, observer bias, responder bias, misclassification*)

Informed consent Voluntary agreement to participate in an epidemiological study after receiving sufficient details of the aims, methods, and potential risks and benefits of the study.

Intention-to-treat analysis In *intervention studies*: subjects are analysed on the basis of initial *intervention allocation* irrespective of whether they complied with this allocation.

Interaction See *effect modification.*

Interim analysis Independent analysis of a *randomized controlled trial* before the planned finish in the case of safety concerns or lack of study *power* to detect an effect.

Internal validity The extent to which differences between comparison groups can be attributed to the association, and not *confounding* or *bias* in the study. (Contrast: *external validity*)

Intervention The preventive or therapeutic measure under study in an *intervention study.* Also, refers to medical or public health involvement to change the developmental process of an *outcome.*

Intervention efficacy A measure of the proportion of incidence of an *outcome* that can be prevented by an *intervention.* (See also *protective efficacy*)

Intervention study *Analytical* study designed to test whether there is a causal relationship by reducing/removing exposure to a *risk factor*, or increasing/introducing exposure to a *protective factor*, and observing the effect on the *outcome.* A *randomized controlled trial* is an example of an intervention study design. (Contrast: *observational study*)

Latent Time between acquiring an *outcome* and appearance of *symptoms.*

Lead-time bias A type of *bias* resulting from the time difference between detection of an *outcome* or *exposure* and the appearance of symptoms, which may lead to an apparent increase in survival time even if there is no effect on the outcome.

Length-time bias A type of *bias* resulting from differences in the length of time taken for an *outcome* to progress to severe effects, which may affect the apparent *efficacy* of a *screening* method.

Life-table Table showing probability of death before next birthday for each age in a population.

Masking See *blinding*.

Matching A technique used to control for *confounding* during study design. The comparison groups are selected to have the same distribution of potential confounders by matching individually (pair matching) or at a group level (frequency matching).

Measurement bias *Information bias* introduced by tools for measuring or assessing the *exposure* or *outcome*.

Minimization Method of *allocation* that aims to minimize differences between the *intervention* and *control* arms in a small *randomized controlled trial* where there may be several *confounders* or *effect modifiers*.

Necessary cause A *component cause* that is essential for an outcome to occur.

Negative predictive value The proportion of individuals identified as not having an *outcome* by a *screening* or diagnostic method that truly do not have the outcome. (See *positive predictive value*, *screening*, *sensitivity*, *specificity*)

Nested case-control study *Case-control study* where *cases* and *controls* are identified from a *prospective cohort* study, reducing problems of *information bias*.

Non-differential misclassification Incorrect classification of *exposure* or *outcome* of study subjects because of *information bias*, where this does not vary between comparison groups. This can lead to an underestimation of the strength (statistical significance) of an association.

Non-inferiority trial A *randomized-controlled trial* which aims to determine that one intervention is no worse than another.

Notifiable disease A disease that is required by law to be reported to government authorities to enable national *surveillance*.

Null hypothesis A falsifiable *hypothesis* against which to statistically test data – usually, that there is no association between an exposure and outcome. (Contrast: *alternative hypothesis*)

Observational study Study in which the role of the investigator is to observe. Can be *descriptive* or *analytical*. *Ecological, cross-sectional, cohort*, and *case-control* are examples of observational analytical study designs. (Contrast: *intervention study*)

Observer bias *Information bias* introduced by those measuring or assessing the *exposure* or *outcome*.

Occupational cohort A group of individuals selected for study based on shared occupation.

Odds (of exposure) The number of individuals in a defined *population* exposed to a risk *factor*, divided by the number of individuals not exposed to that risk factor in the same *population*.

Odds (of outcome) The number of new *cases* of an *outcome* that develop in a defined *population* of individuals at risk during a specified period, divided by the number of individuals who do not develop the outcome during the same time period. It can be interpreted as the ratio of the *risk* that the outcome will occur to the risk that it will not occur during a specified period.

Odds ratio (of exposure) Calculated as the *odds* of *exposure* in those with the outcome, divided by the odds of exposure in those without the outcome. Used in *case-control studies* as an estimate of the *relative risk*, because incidence cannot be measured.

Odds ratio (of outcome) A measure of *relative risk*. Calculated as the *odds* of *outcome* in those exposed, divided by the odds of outcome in those unexposed.

Outbreak A sudden *epidemic*, usually of short duration. (See *epidemic*)

Outcome A health state or event of interest such as infection, illness, disability or death, or a health indicator such as high blood pressure or presence of antibodies. Can also be specified as the opposite of any of these.

Over-diagnosis A type of *bias* resulting from early detection of an *outcome* to progress to severe effects that may affect the apparent *efficacy* of a *screening* method.

Overmatching In a *case-control study*: where *matching* results in *cases* and *controls* that are too similar with respect to the *exposure* of interest to enable detection of an association with *outcome*.

P-value The numerical probability that an observed value or estimated association from a *sample* occurred by chance alone, and that it does not exist in the *population* from which the sample was selected.

Pandemic An *epidemic* that is occurring in populations over many countries or worldwide.

Passive surveillance The *surveillance* of an *outcome* by detection of *cases* when they seek health care.

Per-protocol analysis In *intervention studies*: subjects are analysed on the basis of actual compliance with initial *intervention allocation*.

Period prevalence The number of existing *cases* of an *outcome* in a defined *population* during a specified (short) period of time divided by the total number of people in that *population* during the same time period. It is a *proportion*.

Person-time at risk The sum of the time each individual in a defined population is at risk of an *outcome*. It is used as a denominator in the calculation of *incidence rates*.

Pilot study A small-scale study conducted prior to the main study to test methods, data collection, data entry, etc.

Placebo An inert medication or procedure that may be given to the *control* group in an *intervention trial*, specified as a placebo-controlled trial.

Point prevalence (Synonym: *prevalence*) The number of existing *cases* of an *outcome* in a defined *population* at one point in time divided by the total number of people in that *population* at the same time point. It is a *proportion*.

Population Individuals with a shared characteristic (usually geographic area). (See *general population, sample population, target population*)

Population at risk Individuals who could develop the *outcome* if *exposed*.

Population attributable fraction (Synonym: *population attributable risk percentage*) A measure that calculates the *population attributable risk* as a proportion of the incidence of *outcome* in the population, i.e. the proportion of *cases* in the population that may be due to the *exposure*, and that could be prevented if the exposure were eliminated completely.

Population attributable risk A measure that calculates the additional incidence of *outcome* in the population after subtracting the incidence that would have occurred in the absence of *exposure* (i.e. in those *unexposed*). (See also *attributable risk*)

Population attributable risk percentage See *population attributable fraction*.

Positive predictive value The proportion of individuals identified as having an *outcome* by a *screening* or diagnostic method that truly have the outcome. (See *negative predictive value*, *screening*, *sensitivity*, *specificity*)

Power The statistical probability of detecting an association if it is real.

Precision The statistical probability of detecting an association by chance (i.e. if it is not real).

Prevalence See *point prevalence* and *period prevalence*.

Prevalence ratio A measure of *relative risk*. Calculated as the prevalence of outcome in those exposed to a *risk factor*, divided by the prevalence of outcome in those unexposed.

Preventable fraction A measure that calculates the additional incidence of *outcome* in those *unexposed* to a *protective factor* after subtracting the incidence that would have occurred in the presence of *exposure* (i.e. in those *exposed*). It is calculated by subtracting the relative risk from 1. (Contrast: *attributable fraction*) (See also *protective efficacy*)

Prevention paradox The concept that a measure that brings large population benefits may not benefit all individuals.

Primary prevention *Intervention* to prevent the onset of an *outcome* by removing or reducing *exposure*. (Contrast: *secondary prevention*, *tertiary prevention*)

Probability A measure of the likelihood of an event occurring.

Prognosis A medical term used to describe the likely result (e.g. survival, recovery) of an *outcome*.

Proportion The relationship between two numbers of the same type where one is a part and the other the whole. It can only take values between 0 and 1 (or between 0% and 100% if expressed as a percentage). (See *prevalence*, *risk*)

Prospective cohort A study in which ongoing data collection enables measurement of *outcome* after exposure has been recorded. (Contrast: *retrospective study*)

Protective efficacy A measure of the proportion of incidence of an *outcome* that can be prevented by a *protective factor*. (See also *preventable fraction*)

Protective factor (Synonym: protective *risk factor*) A *risk factor* that is associated with a decreased probability of a negative health *outcome*. (Contrast: *risk factor*)

Random allocation See *randomization*.

Random error The variation of an observed *sample* value from the true *population* value due to *chance* alone.

Random selection Selection in a random (unpredictable) manner where each study unit (person, village, school) has an equal (or known) probability of being selected.

Randomization Where allocation to *intervention* groups is determined by chance, i.e. each study unit has the same probability of being allocated to each of the intervention groups, and the probability that a given unit will receive an intervention is independent of the probability that any other unit will receive the same intervention. (See *randomized controlled trial*)

Randomized controlled trial An *intervention study* in which the *intervention* is compared to a *control*, and allocation of intervention is by *randomization*.

Rate The relationship between two numbers of different types. In epidemiology, it refers to the occurrence of events per unit time. (See *incidence rate*)

Rate difference See *attributable risk*.

Rate ratio See *incidence rate ratio*.

Ratio The relationship between two numbers of the same type, either expressed as *a:b* or *a/b*. (See *prevalence ratio, risk ratio, odds ratio, incidence rate ratio, standardized ratio*)

Reference category The group against which all others are compared. This is usually the *unexposed* group.

Regression *Statistical modelling* to explain how much variation in one variable may be the result of other variables. It enables us to estimate the association between *exposure* and *outcome*, adjusting for the effects of *confounding* and *effect modification*.

Relative risk An estimate of the magnitude of association between *exposure* and incidence of an *outcome*. It can be interpreted as the likelihood of developing an *outcome* in those exposed compared with those unexposed. It can be calculated as *prevalence ratio, risk ratio, odds ratio* or *incidence rate ratio*.

Representative sample A *sample* that has the same characteristics as the *population* from which it was selected.

Residual confounding The effects of *confounding* that remain even after adjustment because data on the *confounder* are not sufficiently accurate.

Responder bias *Information bias* introduced by study participants, or those providing relevant information on study participants.

Restriction A technique used to control for *confounding* during study design. It limits the study to people who are similar in relation to the confounder.

Retrospective cohort study A study in which historical data on *exposure* and *outcome* are collected, and there is no *follow-up* of study participants. (Contrast: *prospective study*)

Reverse causality A situation in which an apparent *risk factor* may be a consequence of the *outcome*.

Risk (Synonym: *cumulative incidence*) The number of new *cases* of an *outcome* that develop in a defined *population* of individuals at risk during a specified period, divided by the total number of individuals at risk during the same period. It is a *proportion* and can be interpreted as the probability that the *outcome* will occur within a specified time.

Risk difference See *attributable risk*.

Risk factor (Synonym: *exposure*) An environmental (e.g. radiation), socio-economic (e.g. occupation), behavioural (e.g. alcohol consumption), physical (e.g. height) or inherited (e.g. blood group) factor associated with an increased probability of a negative health *outcome*. (Contrast: *protective risk factor*)

Risk ratio A measure of *relative risk*. Calculated as the *risk* of *outcome* in those exposed, divided by the risk of outcome in those unexposed.

Sample A subset of a *population* selected for study.

Sample population *Subjects* selected for epidemiological study from a wider *population*. (See *general population*)

Sample size The number of study units (individuals, groups) under study.

Screening The *systematic* detection of an *outcome* or indicators of increased risk for an outcome among apparently healthy people.

Secondary attack rate A specific type of *risk*: the number of new *cases* of an *outcome* that develop among contacts of an initial *case* during a specified period, divided by the total number of contacts at risk during the same period.

Secondary prevention *Intervention* to prevent the development of adverse health consequences of an early stage *outcome*. (Contrast: *primary prevention*, *tertiary prevention*)

Secular trends Changes in the *frequency* of an *outcome* or *exposure* in a *population* over time that are expected to be long-term.

Selection bias Error due to *systematic* differences in characteristics between the study participants and the *population* from which they are selected, or between the groups being compared within the study.

Sensitivity (Synonym: *true positive rate*) The *proportion* of individuals who truly have an *outcome* that are correctly identified by a *screening* or diagnostic method. (Contrast: *specificity*)

Sentinel surveillance The *surveillance* of an *outcome* by detecting *cases* through designated institutions with quality control of diagnosis and reporting.

Specificity (Synonym: *true negative rate*) The *proportion* of individuals who truly do not have an *outcome* that are correctly identified by a *screening* or diagnostic method. (Contrast: *sensitivity*)

Standard population A *population* with a defined structure with respect to a modifying factor such as age, gender, etc.

Standardization (direct) A technique to remove structural differences between populations so that they may be compared. The direct method applies the stratified frequency of outcome in the *study population* to a *standard population* structure to obtain a weighted average.

Standardization (indirect) A technique to remove structural differences between populations so that they may be compared. The indirect method applies the stratified frequency of outcome in a *standard population* to the *study population* structure to obtain the estimated population frequency. This is used to calculate the *standardized ratio*.

Standardized frequency The expected frequency in a population if it had the same structure as a *standard population*, enabling comparison of different populations or time periods. This is obtained by *standardization*. (Contrast: *crude frequency*)

Standardized ratio A comparative measure of the difference in observed and expected *outcome* frequency for a population of interest to enable the comparison of frequency in two populations, adjusting for differences in population structure.

Statistical modelling Definition of the relationship between two variables using mathematical descriptions. (See *regression*)

Statistical significance The probability that a result did not occur by chance. (See *P-value*)

Stratification The process of separating a *sample* into several sub-samples by specified criteria. It can be used to control for *confounding* during analysis, or to detect *effect modification*.

Study population A group of individuals being studied, who may be defined by characteristics such as gender, age, geography, etc.

Study sample A subset of individuals selected for study, usually at random from the *study population*.

Subject An individual or group participating in a study.

Subjects Units of an epidemiological study. These may be, for example, individuals, households, communities, geographical areas or countries.

Sufficient cause A factor or set of factors that inevitably produces the outcome.

Surveillance The monitoring of *outcomes* in a *population* over time.

Survey A method of collecting information to describe something.

Susceptible An individual at risk of acquiring the *outcome* of interest. For example, for many infectious diseases to which immunity is acquired, an immune individual is no longer susceptible (at risk) to infection. This may also apply to individuals with certain genetic characteristics.

Symptoms Changes noticed by a patient indicating the presence of an adverse health *outcome*.

Systematic Method that is non-random, ordered or organized.

Target population The *population* to which the results of an epidemiological study are to be extrapolated, or to which a public health intervention is to be applied. This may be a subset or the whole of the *general population*.

Tertiary prevention *Intervention* to reduce progression of an established *outcome* and prevent complications or more severe consequences. (Contrast: *primary prevention*, *secondary prevention*)

Unexposed Those subjects who have not experienced or do not possess (e.g. genetic or physical characteristics) the *risk factor* of interest.

Vaccine efficacy A measure of the proportion of incidence of an *outcome* that can be prevented by administration of a vaccine. (See also *protective efficacy*)

Washout period Period after an *intervention* has been removed during which its effect declines.

References

Ahmad, O. B., Boschi-Pinto, C., Lopez, A. D., et al. (2001) *Age Standardization of Rates: A new WHO standard*. GPE Discussion Paper Series. Geneva: World Health Organization.

Altman, D. G. and Bland, J. M. (2005) Treatment allocation by minimisation. *British Medical Journal*, 330: 843.

Ascherio, A., Munger, K. L., Lennette, E. T., et al. (2001) Epstein-Barr virus antibodies and risk of multiple sclerosis: a prospective study. *Journal of the American Medical Association*, 286: 3083–8.

Aylin, P., Alexandrescu, R., Jen, M. H., et al. (2013) Day of week of procedure and 30 day mortality for elective surgery: retrospective analysis of hospital episode statistics. *British Medical Journal*, 346: f2424.

Bastawrous, A., Rono, H. K., Livingstone, I. A., et al. (2015) Development and validation of a smartphone-based visual acuity test (Peek Acuity) for clinical practice and community-based fieldwork. *Journal of the American Medical Association Ophthalmology*, 133: 930–7.

Bauer, A. Z. and Kriebel, D. (2013) Prenatal and perinatal analgesic exposure and autism: an ecological link. *Environmental Health*, 12: 41.

Becher, H. (1992) The concept of residual confounding in regression models and some applications. *Statistics in Medicine*, 11: 1747–58.

Bhatt, A. (2010) Evolution of clinical research: a history before and beyond James Lind. *Perspectives in Clinical Research*, 1: 6–10.

Bobak, M. and Leon, D. A. (1999) Pregnancy outcomes and outdoor air pollution: an ecological study in districts of the Czech Republic 1986–8. *Occupational and Environmental Medicine*, 56: 539–43.

Bonaventure, A., Harewood, R., Stiller, C. A., et al. (2017) Worldwide comparison of survival from childhood leukaemia for 1995–2009, by subtype, age, and sex (CONCORD-2): a population-based study of individual data for 89,828 children from 198 registries in 53 countries. *Lancet Haematology*, 4: e202–17.

Boston University (2016) *Framingham Heart Study: Research milestones* [Online]. National Heart, Lung, and Blood Institute and Boston University. Available at: https://www.framinghamheartstudy.org/about-fhs/research-milestones.php [Accessed 22 September 2016].

Bouvard, V., Loomis, D., Guyton, K. Z., et al. (2015) Carcinogenicity of consumption of red and processed meat. *Lancet Oncology*, 16: 1599–600.

Brasil, P., Pereira, J. P., Jr., Moreira, M. E., et al. (2016) Zika virus infection in pregnant women in Rio de Janeiro. *New England Journal of Medicine*, 375: 2321–34.

Brown, C. A. and Lilford, R. J. (2006) The stepped wedge trial design: a systematic review. *BioMed Central Medical Research Methodology*, 6: 54.

Cao-Lormeau, V. M., Blake, A., Mons, S., et al. (2016) Guillain-Barré syndrome outbreak associated with Zika virus infection in French Polynesia: a case-control study. *Lancet*, 387: 1531–9.

Cauchemez, S., Besnard, M., Bompard, P., et al. (2016) Association between Zika virus and microcephaly in French Polynesia, 2013–15: a retrospective study. *Lancet*, 387: 2125–32.

Centers for Disease Control and Prevention (1999) Healthier mothers and babies. *Morbidity and Mortality Weekly Report*, 48: 849–50.

Centers for Disease Control and Prevention (2009) Estimated county-level prevalence of diabetes and obesity – United States, 2007. *Morbidity Mortality Weekly Report*, 58: 1259–63.

Centers for Disease Control and Prevention (2010) Summary of notifiable disease – United States, 2008. *Morbidity and Mortality Weekly Report*, 57: 1–94.

Centers for Disease Control and Prevention (2011) Increased transmission and outbreaks of measles – European region, 2011. *Morbidity and Mortality Weekly Report*, 60: 1605–10.

Centers for Disease Control and Prevention (2017a) *Sexually Transmitted Disease Morbidity for Selected STDs by Age, Race/Ethnicity and Gender 1996–2014* [Online]. Available at: http://wonder.cdc.gov/std-race-age.html [Accessed 15 May 2017].

Centers for Disease Control and Prevention (2017b) *Transparent Reporting of Evaluations with Nonrandomized Designs (TREND)* [Online]. Available at: https://www.cdc.gov/trendstatement [Accessed 22 May 2017].

Chow, A., Ho, H., Win, M.-K. and Leo, Y.-S. (2017) Assessing sensitivity and specificity of surveillance case definitions for Zika virus disease. *Emerging Infectious Diseases*, 23: 677–9.

Cisse, B., Ba, E. H., Sokhna, C., et al. (2016) Effectiveness of seasonal malaria chemoprevention in children under 10 years of age in Senegal: a stepped-wedge cluster-randomised trial. *PLoS Medicine*, 13: e1002175.

Colau, J. C., Vincent, S., Marijnen, P., et al. (2012) Efficacy of a non-hormonal treatment, BRN-01, on menopausal hot flashes: a multicenter, randomized, double-blind, placebo-controlled trial. *Drugs in R&D*, 12: 107–19.

CONSORT Group (2010) *The CONSORT Statement* [Online]. Available at: http://www.consort-statement.org [Accessed 22 May 2017].

Costello, A., Dua, T., Duran, P., et al. (2016) Defining the syndrome associated with congenital Zika virus infection. *Bulletin of the World Health Organization*, 94: 406–406A.

Coughlin, S. S. (2006) Ethical issues in epidemiologic research and public health practice. *Emerging Themes in Epidemiology*, 3: 16.

Cramer, J. D., Fu, P., Harth, K. C., et al. (2010) Analysis of the rising incidence of thyroid cancer using the Surveillance, Epidemiology and End Results national cancer data registry. *Surgery*, 148: 1147–52; discussion 1152–3.

Cutts, F. T., Zaman, S. M., Enwere, G., et al. (2005) Efficacy of nine-valent pneumococcal conjugate vaccine against pneumonia and invasive pneumococcal disease in The Gambia: randomised, double-blind, placebo-controlled trial. *Lancet*, 365: 1139–46.

Day, L., Fildes, B., Gordon, I., et al. (2002) Randomised factorial trial of falls prevention among older people living in their own homes. *British Medical Journal*, 325: 128.

De Araujo, T. V., Rodrigues, L. C., De Alencar Ximenes, R. A., et al. (2016) Association between Zika virus infection and microcephaly in Brazil, January to May, 2016: preliminary report of a case-control study. *Lancet Infectious Diseases*, 16: 1356–63.

Di Forti, M., Marconi, A., Carra, E., et al. (2015) Proportion of patients in south London with first-episode psychosis attributable to use of high potency cannabis: a case-control study. *Lancet Psychiatry*, 2: 233–8.

Doll, R. and Hill, A. B. (1950) Smoking and carcinoma of the lung: preliminary report. *British Medical Journal*, 2: 739–48.

Doll, R. and Peto, R. (1976) Mortality in relation to smoking: 20 years' observations on male British doctors. *British Medical Journal*, 2: 1525–36.

Doll, R., Gray, R., Hafner, B., et al. (1980) Mortality in relation to smoking: 22 years' observations on female British doctors. *British Medical Journal*, 280: 967–71.

Durand, M. A. and Chantler, T. (eds.) (2014) *Principles of Social Research* (2nd edn.). Maidenhead: Open University Press.

Dwan, K., Gamble, C., Williamson, P. R., et al. (2013) Systematic review of the empirical evidence of study publication bias and outcome reporting bias – an updated review. *PLoS One*, 8: e66844.

Elmore, J. G. and Feinstein, A. R. (1994) Joseph Goldberger: an unsung hero of American clinical epidemiology. *Annals of Internal Medicine*, 121: 372–5.

Emberson, J., Whincup, P., Morris, R., et al. (2004) Evaluating the impact of population and high-risk strategies for the primary prevention of cardiovascular disease. *European Heart Journal*, 25: 484–91.

Fletcher, A., Cragg, L. and Kazi, A. (2013) The Rose hypothesis: advantages of whole population over targeted approaches, in L. Cragg, M. Davies and W. MacDowall (eds.) *Health Promotion Theory* (2nd edn.). Maidenhead: Open University Press.

Fontanet, A. L., Messele, T., Dejene, A., et al. (1998) Age- and sex-specific HIV-1 prevalence in the urban community setting of Addis Ababa, Ethiopia. *AIDS*, 12: 315–22.

Franca, G. V., Schuler-Faccini, L., Oliveira, W. K., et al. (2016) Congenital Zika virus syndrome in Brazil: a case series of the first 1501 livebirths with complete investigation. *Lancet*, 388: 891–7.

Freedman, N. D., Park, Y., Abner, C. C., et al. (2012) Association of coffee drinking with total and cause-specific mortality. *New England Journal of Medicine*, 366: 1891–1904.

Gay, N., Rousset, D., Huc, P., et al. (2016) Seroprevalence of Asian lineage Chikungunya virus infection on Saint Martin Island, 7 months after the 2013 emergence. *American Journal of Tropical Medicine and Hygiene*, 94: 393–6.

GBD 2015 DALYs and HALE Collaborators (2016) Global, regional, and national disability-adjusted life-years (DALYs) for 315 diseases and injuries and healthy life expectancy (HALE), 1990–2015: a systematic analysis for the Global Burden of Disease Study 2015. *Lancet*, 388: 1603–58.

GBD 2015 Mortality and Causes of Death Collaborators (2016) Global, regional, and national life expectancy, all-cause mortality, and cause-specific mortality for 249 causes of death, 1980–2015: a systematic analysis for the Global Burden of Disease Study 2015. *Lancet*, 388, 1459–544.

Grimes, D.A. and Schultz, K.F. (2002) An overview of clinical research, the lay of the land. *The Lancet*, 359: 57–61

Hanson, K., Nathan, R., Marchant, T., et al. (2008) Vouchers for scaling up insecticide-treated nets in Tanzania: methods for monitoring and evaluation of a national health system intervention. *BioMed Central Public Health*, 8: 205.

Hayes, R. J. and Moulton, L. H. (2009) *Cluster Randomised Trials*. Boca Raton, FL: Chapman & Hall/CRC Press.

Henao-Restrepo, A. M., Camacho, A., Longini, I. M., et al. (2017) Efficacy and effectiveness of an rVSV-vectored vaccine in preventing Ebola virus disease: final results from the Guinea ring vaccination, open-label, cluster-randomised trial (Ebola Ça Suffit!). *Lancet*, 389: 505–18.

Henderson, D. A. (1987) Principles and lessons from the smallpox eradication programme. *Bulletin of the World Health Organization*, 65: 535–46.

Hill, A. B. (1965) The environment and disease: association or causation? *Proceedings of the Royal Society of Medicine*, 58: 295–300.

Hippocrates (2015) On airs, waters and places, in *Complete Works of Hippocrates.* Hastings: Delphi Classics.

Honjo, K. (2004) Social epidemiology: definition, history, and research examples. *Environmental Health and Preventive Medicine*, 9: 193–9.

Imamura, F., O'Connor, L., Ye, Z., et al. (2015) Consumption of sugar sweetened beverages, artificially sweetened beverages, and fruit juice and incidence of type 2 diabetes: systematic review, meta-analysis, and estimation of population attributable fraction. *British Medical Journal*, 351: h3576.

Janssen, H. C., Samson, M. M. and Verhaar, H. J. (2002) Vitamin D deficiency, muscle function, and falls in elderly people. *American Journal of Clinical Nutrition*, 75: 611–15.

Johnson, A. P. (2015) Surveillance of antibiotic resistance. *Philosophical Transactions of the Royal Society of London B: Biological Sciences*, 370: 20140080.

Jones, C., Abeku, T. A., Rapuoda, B., et al. (2008) District-based malaria epidemic early warning systems in East Africa: perceptions of acceptability and usefulness among key staff at health facility, district and central levels. *Social Science and Medicine*, 67: 292–300.

Kaprio, J. (2000) Science, medicine and the future: genetic epidemiology. *British Medical Journal*, 320: 1257–9.

Khoury, M. J. and Beaty, T. H. (1994) Applications of the case-control method in genetic epidemiology. *Epidemiologic Reviews*, 16: 134–50.

Kindhauser, M. K., Allen, T., Frank, V., et al. (2016) Zika: the origin and spread of a mosquito-borne virus. *Bulletin of the World Health Organization*, 94: 675–686C.

Kirkwood, B. R. and Sterne, J. A. C. (2003) *Essential Medical Statistics*. Oxford: Blackwell Science.

Krieger, N. (2003) Genders, sexes, and health: what are the connections – and why does it matter? *International Journal of Epidemiology*, 32: 652–7.

Kuh, D., Ben-Shlomo, Y., Lynch, J., et al. (2003) Life course epidemiology. *Journal of Epidemiology and Community Health*, 57: 778–83.

Lilienfeld, D. E. (2007) Celebration: William Farr (1807–1883) – an appreciation on the 200th anniversary of his birth. *International Journal of Epidemiology*, 36: 985–7.

Maganga, G. D., Kapetshi, J., Berthet, N., et al. (2014) Ebola virus disease in the Democratic Republic of Congo. *New England Journal of Medicine*, 371: 2083–91.

Marcus, P. M., Bergstralh, E. J., Fagerstrom, R. M., et al. (2000) Lung cancer mortality in the Mayo Lung Project: impact of extended follow-up. *Journal of the National Cancer Institute*, 92: 1308–16.

Matthews, T. J., MacDorman, M. F. and Thoma, M. E. (2015) Infant mortality statistics from the 2013 period linked birth/infant death data set. *National Vital Statistics Reports*, 64: 1–30.

Menafricar, C. (2015) The diversity of meningococcal carriage across the African meningitis belt and the impact of vaccination with a group A meningococcal conjugate vaccine. *Journal of Infectious Diseases*, 212: 1298–307.

Morabia, A. (1996) P.C.A. Louis and the birth of clinical epidemiology. *Journal of Clinical Epidemiology*, 49: 1327–33.

Moss, A. R., Osmond, D., Bacchetti, P., et al. (1987) Risk factors for AIDS and HIV seropositivity in homosexual men. *American Journal of Epidemiology*, 125: 1035–47.

Mounts, A. W., Kwong, H., Izurieta, H. S., et al. (1999) Case-control study of risk factors for avian influenza A (H5N1) disease, Hong Kong, 1997. *Journal of Infectious Diseases*, 180: 505–8.

Murray, C. J. L. and Lopez, A. D. (eds.) (1996) *The Global Burden of Disease: A comprehensive assessment of mortality and disability from diseases, injuries, and risk factors in 1990 and projected to 2020*. Boston, MA: Harvard School of Public Health.

Nadkarni, A., Weobong, B., Weiss, H. A., et al. (2017) Counselling for Alcohol Problems (CAP), a lay counsellor-delivered brief psychological treatment for harmful drinking in men, in primary care in India: a randomised controlled trial. *Lancet*, 389: 186–95.

Otsuka, R., Yatsuya, H. and Tamakoshi, K. (2014) Descriptive epidemiological study of food intake among Japanese adults: analyses by age, time and birth cohort model. *BioMed Central Public Health,* 14: 328.

Pan American Health Organization (2017) *Zika – Epidemiological update*. Washington, DC: Pan American Health Organization/World Health Organization.

Pealing, L., Wing, K., Mathur, R., et al. (2015) Risk of tuberculosis in patients with diabetes: population based cohort study using the UK clinical practice research datalink. *BioMed Central Medicine*, 13: 135–50.

Penman, A. D. and Johnson, W. D. (2006) The changing shape of the body mass index distribution curve in the population: implications for public health policy to reduce the prevalence of adult obesity. *Preventing Chronic Disease*, 3: A74.

Pillai, A., Patel, V., Cardozo, P., et al. (2008) Non-traditional lifestyles and prevalence of mental disorders in adolescents in Goa, India. *British Journal of Psychiatry*, 192: 45–51.

Pisa, D., Alonso, R., Rodal, I., et al. (2015) Different brain regions are infected with fungi in Alzheimer's disease. *Scientific Reports*, 5: 15015.

Plummer, M., De Martel, C., Vignat, J., et al. (2016) Global burden of cancers attributable to infections in 2012: a synthetic analysis. *Lancet Global Health*, 4: e609–16.

Porta, M. S. and International Epidemiological Association (eds.) (2008) *A Dictionary of Epidemiology*. Oxford: Oxford University Press.

Ramazzini, B. (2001) Voices from the past: diseases of workers. *American Journal of Public Health*, 91: 1380–2.

Ramsay, M. E. (2013) Measles: the legacy of low vaccine coverage. *Archives of Disease in Childhood*, 98: 752–4.

Rasmussen, S. A., Jamieson, D. J., Honein, M. A., et al. (2016) Zika virus and birth defects – reviewing the evidence for causality. *New England Journal of Medicine*, 374: 1981–7.

Richards, T. (1983) Farr sighted. *British Medical Journal*, 286: 1736–7.

Rim, S. H., Joseph, D. A., Steele, C. B., et al. (2011) Colorectal cancer screening – United States, 2002, 2004, 2006, and 2008. *Morbidity and Mortality Weekly Report*, 60: 42–6.

Roberts, I., Shakur, H., Afolabi, A., et al. (2011) The importance of early treatment with tranexamic acid in bleeding trauma patients: an exploratory analysis of the CRASH-2 randomised controlled trial. *Lancet*, 377: 1096–101, 1101.e1–2.

Ronsmans, C., Chowdhury, M. E., Dasgupta, S. K., et al. (2010) Effect of parent's death on child survival in rural Bangladesh: a cohort study. *Lancet*, 375: 2024–31.

Rose, G. (1992) *The Strategy of Preventive Medicine*. Oxford: Oxford University Press.

Rothman, K. J. (1996) Lessons from John Graunt. *Lancet*, 347: 37–9.

Rothman, K. J. and Greenland, S. (2005) Causation and causal inference in epidemiology. *American Journal of Public Health*, 95: S144–50.

Schatzkin, A., Piantadosi, S., Miccozzi, M., et al. (1989) Alcohol consumption and breast cancer: a cross-national correlation study. *International Journal of Epidemiology*, 18: 28–31.

Schuchat, A., Bell, B. P. and Redd, S. C. (2011) The science behind preparing and responding to pandemic influenza: the lessons and limits of science. *Clinical Infectious Diseases*, 52 (suppl. 1): S8–12.

Schulz, K. F. and Grimes, D. A. (2002) Case-control studies: research in reverse. *Lancet*, 359: 431–4.

Snow, J. (1936) *On the Mode of Communication of Cholera (being a reprint of two papers)*. London: Oxford University Press.

The Gambia Hepatitis Study Group (1987) The Gambia Hepatitis Intervention Study. *Cancer Research*, 47: 5782–7.

Tsang, C. and Cromwell, D. (eds.) (2017) *Health Care Evaluation*. London: Open University Press.

United Nations (2015a) *Transforming Our World: 2030 agenda for sustainable development* [Online]. Available at: https://sustainabledevelopment.un.org/content/documents/21252030%20Agenda% 20for%20Sustainable%20Development%20web.pdf [Accessed 22 May 2017].

United Nations (2015b) *World Population Prospects: The 2015 revision* [Online]. Available at: https:// esa.un.org/unpd/wpp/ [Accessed 20 April 2017].

Victora, C. G., Habicht, J. P. and Bryce, J. (2004) Evidence-based public health: moving beyond randomized trials. *American Journal of Public Health*, 94: 400–5.

Wacker, C., Prkno, A., Brunkhorst, F. M., et al. (2013) Procalcitonin as a diagnostic marker for sepsis: a systematic review and meta-analysis. *Lancet Infectious Diseases*, 13: 426–35.

Wakefield, A. J., Murch, S. H., Anthony, A., et al. (1998) Ileal-lymphoid-nodular hyperplasia, non-specific colitis, and pervasive developmental disorder in children. *Lancet*, 351: 637–41.

Weinstock, M. A., Colditz, G. A., Willett, W. C., et al. (1991) Recall (report) bias and reliability in the retrospective assessment of melanoma risk. *American Journal of Epidemiology*, 133: 240–5.

Weiss, H. A., Quigley, M. A. and Hayes, R. J. (2000) Male circumcision and risk of HIV infection in Sub-Saharan Africa: a systematic review and meta-analysis. *AIDS*, 14: 2361–70.

Weiss, N. S. (2002) Can the 'specificity' of an association be rehabilitated as a basis for supporting a causal hypothesis? *Epidemiology*, 13: 6–8.

Westerlund, H., Vahtera, J., Ferrie, J. E., et al. (2010) Effect of retirement on major chronic conditions and fatigue: French GAZEL occupational cohort study. *British Medical Journal*, 341: c6149.

Wilson, J. M. and Jungner, Y. G. (1968) *Principles and Practice of Screening for Disease*. Public Health Papers. Geneva: World Health Organization.

Winkelstein, W. (2006) Janet Elizabeth Lane-Claypon: a forgotten epidemiologic pioneer. *Epidemiology*, 17: 705.

World Health Organization (2005) *International Health Regulations* [Online]. Available at: http://www.who.int/topics/international_health_regulations/en/ [Accessed 22 May 2017].

World Health Organization (2008) *The World Health Report 2008: Primary Health Care – Now more than ever*. Geneva: World Health Organization.

World Health Organization (2014) *WHO Guidelines for Indoor Air Quality: Household fuel combustion*. Geneva: World Health Organization.

World Health Organization (2015) *Guideline: Sugars intake for adults and children*. Geneva: World Health Organization.

World Health Organization (2016a) *Ambient Pollution: A global assessment of exposure and burden of disease*. Geneva: World Health Organization.

World Health Organization (2016b) *Cancer Mortality Database* [Online]. Available at: http://www-dep.iarc.fr/WHOdb/WHOdb.htm [Accessed 22 February 2017].

World Health Organization (2016c) *El Niño and Health: Global overview*. Geneva: World Health Organization.

World Health Organization (2016d) *Health Policy* [Online]. Available at: http://www.who.int/topics/health_policy/en/ [Accessed 17 November 2016].

World Health Organization (2017a) *Global Health Observatory* [Online]. Available at: http://www.who.int/gho/about/en/ [Accessed 22 May 2017].

World Health Organization (2017b) *Global Outbreak Alert and Response Network* [Online]. Available at: https://extranet.who.int/goarn/ [Accessed 22 May 2017].

World Medical Association (2013) *WMA Declaration of Helsinki – Ethical principles for medical research involving human subjects* [Online]. Available at: https://www.wma.net/policies-post/wma-declaration-of-helsinki-ethical-principles-for-medical-research-involving-human-subjects/ [Accessed 22 May 2017].

Zanluca, C., Melo, V. C., Mosimann, A. L., et al. (2015) First report of autochthonous transmission of Zika virus in Brazil. *Memorias do Instituto Oswaldo Cruz*, 110: 569–72.

Index